HEALING HACKS

HEALING HACKS

Bring Your Body
Back to Nature

IAN HART

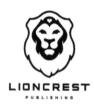

LIONCREST
PUBLISHING

HEALING HACKS
Bring Your Body Back to Nature

ISBN 978-1-5445-0561-9 *Hardcover*
      978-1-5445-0559-6 *Paperback*
      978-1-5445-0560-2 *Ebook*

This book is dedicated to my whole family, and specifically my children, Roman Lion Hart and Zen Saoirse Hart. Your body is a miracle created by God. It is a masterpiece, a perfectly engineered healing machine when given what God intended for it: love, sunlight, nature, movement, oxygen, live food, and when needed, fasting, cleansing, rest, and recovery. I love you all.

CONTENTS

FOREWORD

BY WIM HOF

My name is Wim Hof, "the Iceman." That's the name they gave me after going on numerous challenges into the extremes of nature—the cold, the heat, the height. I used the cold as a tool to jump into my physiology; it gave me a drive to go deeply within. My willingness to go into the unknown made me able to do seemingly impossible things. I climbed Mount Everest into the death zone in shorts. I ran a half marathon barefoot in the arctic circle in midwinter in shorts as well. I ran a full marathon in the desert without drinking water. I hung by one finger on a rope strung between two hot air balloons a mile high in the air and climbed between them.

As I showed these feats and so many more to the world, television crews came in to challenge me. I set twenty-six world records for these stunts, and when I had several disciplines done, I caught the eye of the scientific community. "What this man is doing is not humanly possible," they said, "but he *is* doing it. Let's experiment on him." And that's what they did.

What they found out is that nature is able to teach us to

awaken and control deeply forgotten and lost physiology. Contrary to the historical ideas of medicine and physiology, they found I was able to influence the autonomic nervous system, and with that the endocrine system, and the innate immune system. The Iceman, they saw, was able to go far deeper into the autonomic nervous system, endocrine system, and innate immune system than ever thought possible by science. This changed their perspective. Next, the scientific community wondered if I would be able to pass on my abilities to a group of people, and that's what I did.

Through comparative studies, we showed that everyone actually is able to influence these systems, in a very short period of time, through training in gradual cold exposure, specific breathing exercises, and mindset.

In this book, Ian Hart shows it is possible to find a new experience within yourself by experiencing this connection. By going far deeper within yourself, you can control wherever you are and whatever you've got. Is it Lyme disease? Arthritis? Depression? The specific condition does not matter. Your perspective will be shifted by going deeper.

To develop this knowledge, Ian Hart has followed his heart and his ability to understand by feeling. He went to all kinds of institutions, doctors, and therapies and found this method. He found me, and I found my method in nature. Together we bring this natural ability back to people, so that they can control systems far deeper in themselves than they ever thought possible. That's what this book is all about. You'd better read it and get on your horse, because this is going to be a ride.

INTRODUCTION

"The wound is the place where the light enters you."

—RUMI

I was standing in line at the pharmacy, about to purchase a medication that was going cost me $1,800 a month. The doctor said I'd be on this medication for the rest of my life. The Mayo Clinic website claimed this medication, Entocort, was only effective about 50 percent of the time for my condition.[1]

I was 29 years old and incredibly sick. During my hospital stay, the doctor had rattled off a complicated diagnosis: I was told I had Crohn's disease, had developed ulcers as a result, and that my intestines were twisted. Something in my bloodwork indicated I had been close to death. He said I would never heal fully and that I would have to manage my symptoms with this expensive medication. My health insurance coverage was, in a word, catastrophic. It wasn't going to cover any of this.

---

1   Sarah O'Donnell and Colm A. O'Morain, "Therapeutic Benefits Of Budesonide In Gastroenterology," *Therapeutic Advances in Chronic Disease*, July 2010, 1(4): 177-186.

At the hospital, they'd fed me coffee, pancakes, bacon, Jell-O—all the worst possible foods you could put in a body in gastrointestinal distress. At the same time, they were considering cutting out pieces of my intestines. I knew that wasn't the right environment for healing.

Just after being discharged from the hospital and dropping off the astronomically expensive prescription at the pharmacy window, I broke into tears—both from the state I'd wound up in, and from morphine and Dilaudid withdrawal. They'd pumped both into me in the hospital because the pain was unbelievably excruciating. I hadn't slept for days. I was confused about what to do next.

Entocort is an immunosuppressant, designed to reduce inflammation in the area of the bowel affected by Crohn's disease. The side effects of Entocort can be numerous and severe: inflammation of the liver, nausea, and vomiting, just to name a few of a long list. Since the drug suppresses the immune system, the body becomes less effective at fighting off viruses and even cancer. Once I was on this drug long term, I learned, getting off it would be difficult. Some patients become steroid-dependent and are unable to come off the drug without symptoms flaring. Others become steroid-resistant and are unable to stay symptom-free with the same dose.[2]

I talked to my girlfriend at the time (now the mother of my children) and told her what I'd found out about the drug. We tried to figure out what to do. My mind whirred. *What's*

---

[2] "Corticosteroids and Inflammatory Bowel Disease (IBD)," *IBD Clinical and Research Centre*, 2017.

going on? What's wrong with me? How did I end up in this position? How could I be so sick at such a young age?

Just a few years earlier, my picture had been inside two issues of *Men's Health* magazine as an expert veteran personal trainer. *Men's Health* was putting on a major race they called the Urbanathlon, and I'd created specific training programs for the race that were featured in the magazine. At 26, I'd been in the best shape of my life. Fast forward a year and a half, and the intensity of my symptoms increased until I found myself doubled over on the floor of my apartment in agony. My girlfriend (now wife) took me to the emergency room, where I was hospitalized with a twisted gut, among other life-threatening issues.

Now as I inched closer to the prescription counter, I was caught in a do-or-die moment. I was gripped by fear from what I'd been told by the medical community. *What do I do? Do I get this medication, or not?* My gut said no. Some voice in my head was saying, "*You can heal this. You have to believe.*"

Still standing in line, I called a friend of mine, Dr. Peter Osborne.

"This is what the medical community wants," he said. "They want you to believe you need medication, and that you can't heal yourself. They want you on a drug for the rest of your life. I'm not telling you not to do it—you have to do what you feel is right for you. But there are ways to heal your body. You can heal it naturally."

His words rang true for me and gave credence to that voice in my head that told me I could heal without the drug. I didn't want this prescription—but I'd been standing in line because I was afraid. I had almost died, and the fear that I could end up in an extreme medical crisis yet again was overwhelming. This phone call was the final shift. I hung up the phone, stepped out of line, and never went back to that doctor again.

In fact, I never went back to the allopathic medical community at all. Instead, I started my own healing journey and sought help through holistic means.

The story of how my health spiraled downhill, so far and so fast, is the focus of the first chapter of this book. In my journey to heal, I researched and tested on myself every holistic healing method I could find. I no longer relied on the medical community to manage my symptoms. Instead, I reconnected with myself, trusted in my own experience, and listened to my body to find the best methods to allow it to heal. If you are suffering, you have the potential to do the same.

In the 11 years that I've been on this healing journey, there have been massive strides in holistic approaches to healing and new insights on the mind-body connection. I've been a sponge, spending countless hours studying all this information, testing new practices for myself, and interviewing with hundreds of some of the world's leading healers.

As a health and fitness expert with years of experience, knowledge, and certifications, already the creator of an internationally successful natural back pain relief program, this journey took me to a whole new level of understanding and healing. I built a retreat in a Costa Rican treehouse community to help begin my healing as well as help others heal. I traveled all over the world to learn from experts. I became a certified Wim Hof instructor and practiced breathing techniques, cold exposure, and mindset changes. I began teaching these techniques at my training facilities and seeing what worked best. Along the way, I have spent well over a half a million dollars experimenting with every healing method I could find.

This book is the culmination of everything I've learned so far boiled down to the bare essentials, the most valuable "hacks." It's been an amazing journey with ups and downs, but I've managed to get my wellness and my life back. Considering the dire health crisis that began this journey, recovering my health has been a miracle. I have learned we all have the ability to heal and I am grateful for the challenges that have been thrown my way. As the journey continues, I have a deep sense of gratitude for the path I have gone down, however difficult it has been, and my goal is to transfer this experience and knowledge to you so that you may enhance your health and improve your life.

BACK TO NATURE

I'm not the only person in an extremely dire situation to be told by the medical community there was no way I would heal. Even if your healing journey hasn't involved a hospital visit, you've likely been told that any dis-ease you feel, from a debilitating illness to back pain or the common cold, needs mainstream medical intervention and medication to keep you functioning. Many times, this idea that we require medical assistance to get back to health is flat-out false.

Mainstream medicine has its place, particularly for life-threatening traumatic injuries and critical situations where you're about to die. I am grateful to be living in a society that has made amazing strides in health sciences. When I tore my pec muscle from the bone a few years ago jumping off a cliff in Costa Rica, for example, I was grateful to the surgeons who reattached my tendons to the bone. But much of the dis-ease we experience isn't from traumatic injury. It's from our lifestyles and the habits that have pulled us out of our natural state of health.

At my transformation center, I hear the same stories almost every day: "I used to feel great," clients say. "I had tons of energy. I used to be in shape, and over the years I've lost all my energy. I feel aches and pains all the time. My memory is foggy and I struggle to focus my attention." They describe gastrointestinal issues from bloating to acid reflux. Often, new clients have issues with their digestion, blood pressure, cholesterol—the list goes on and on. This may be a common experience, but it's not normal. I recently looked at a picture of a crowd of Americans at the beach in the 70s and there was not one overweight person in it. Nowadays, the majority of Americans are overweight, out of shape, and unhealthy. It is a sign that the body has been disconnected from what it needs to function optimally, and on the inverse, the body has probably been given substances and exposed to stressors that are breaking it down faster, causing rapid aging and deterioration, both mentally and physically. These symptoms are signs that the body has been disconnected from nature.

HACKING HEALTH

The word "hack" got its modern definition from the members of the MIT Model Railroad Club, who used the word to describe an unusual solution to a complex problem.

Today, it's used to describe clever approaches to a variety of problems, from computer processes to biological systems. "Biohacking" involves solutions or shortcuts for physiological issues—for example, if someone has a hard time sleeping, there are "hacks" to improve sleep quality.

These hacks usually entail some technique to bring us back to our natural state of being. Take blue-blocking glasses, for example. They're designed to reduce our unnatural exposure to the blue light that's not as common in the natural world as it is on our devices and the lights in our houses.

The hacks in this book are techniques I've learned to help us reconnect to nature. Much of the information in this book is an assimilation of ideas I've accrued over a decade of research and experimentation with my own body. Pair the hacks in this book with the healing philosophies of the hackers who teach them, and you will redefine what it means to be healthy, get back in touch with yourself, and return to harmony with nature. All the signs are there; we just need to listen, follow our intuition, and give the body what it needs—and the body will do the rest.

HEALING MYSELF, HEALING OTHERS

Being in the hospital was one of the lowest points of my life. It was hell on earth, and there were times I wanted to end it—it often seemed easier to die than to live with the pain and misery. The life I had was no longer enjoyable. For two years leading up to my hospitalization, every day was a struggle, and every day I was in pain. Things looked even more dire when I ended up in the hospital. But instead of giving up while in the hospital, I made a commitment to myself that I was going to get better, and that when I did, I would share my knowledge with the world to help other suffering people who needed healing. In a way, that was my only option to motivate myself to dig myself out of the darkness I was in. My pain was made bearable by the thought of being able to save or help other people. It gave me hope that something good could come from it.

As I learned the practices that helped my own healing, I shared these hacks with the clients in my training facility, called EarthFIT Mind-Body Transformation Center and online. I started EarthFIT in a 700-square-foot facility in 2009, and it has since expanded five times to 15,000-square-feet across three locations. I also co-founded Back Pain Relief4Life, a program that has helped thousands of people in more than one hundred countries end their back pain in the simplest and most effective way, fast and naturally, without any gadgets or devices. As I worked with all these healing tools with clients, I learned what works quickly, safely, and efficiently and saw amazing transformations in people's health.

Many people come to our programs feeling lost. They're not as energetic or strong as they once were, they don't know how to recover their health, and they're often unable to play the sports they love and do the hobbies or activities they enjoy. As such, they adopt self-limiting beliefs about their abilities, body, and health.

If you picked up this book because you're not performing at your best or you're sick, fatigued, and feel dis-ease, you're not alone. Not only have I been there, but there are many people out there just like you. What I find in today's society is that the majority of the population is lost, confused, distracted, disconnected, and lacks clarity on how to get and maintain *true* health and happiness. In the first chapter of this book, I'll share my own story of the limiting beliefs I held as my health spiraled out of control, and how I shifted my mindset toward one of true healing.

Our environment, thoughts, and feelings govern our energy and our actions. Every healing journey begins with understanding the current state of your mental, physical, and emotional health, as well as the health of your beliefs. In chapter two, we'll take a look at the effect our intentions have on shaping our wellbeing. This can many times have the most powerful influence on our healing.

In the remaining chapters, we'll look at practices and hacks for improving specific areas of health. We can reduce inflammation, improve our stress response and our immune system with breathwork alone, as you'll see in chapter three. Movement plays a vital role in healing, not only for the strength of our muscles, bones, and joints, but for the regulation of our blood sugar, inflammation, and immune response as well. In chapter four, you'll find specific movement programs to target these benefits. Chapters five and six will tackle the complexity of our gut health: we'll see how nutrition and cleansing influence all our body's systems. Spending time in nature holds a variety of benefits for bodies and minds, as you'll see in chapter seven. Lastly, in chapter eight, I'll share how experiences with psychedelics have helped myself and others rewire our body, brains, and beliefs and help spark powerful healing—practices all backed by science.

Ultimately, the body is a beautiful healing machine, and we

can learn how to give it what it needs to heal. In each chapter of this book, we'll look at the work of renowned healers across the world and break down specific techniques to target systems in the body and bring them back to maximum performance.

The heart automatically pumps. A cut automatically heals. Animals don't check their blood pressure, take cholesterol medication, or inject themselves with vaccines. They eat natural, indigenous foods, and move consistently. They're in harmony with nature. Remember you were once a cell that grew into a human without you doing anything. Our bodies, too, can do amazing things when we get out of our own way, remove unnatural toxins and poisons, provide them with what they need, and let them heal automatically. Making this shift back to nature doesn't just require us to change our habits and our actions. We often have to shift our mindset and our belief systems, to connect back to our bodies and believe that we can heal.

My story began with a health crisis that finally made me realize I needed healing and harmonizing, and it was hard to believe I could heal from that dark place. Each step since then has brought me better health and performance, and now I am excited to share that with you, because what you learn in this book may dramatically transform your life.

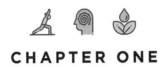

CHAPTER ONE

BACK FROM THE BRINK OF DEATH

One of the hardest decisions I've ever made in my life was to decline my commission as an officer from the Marine Corps at age 26. I had no idea what I would do with my life if I wasn't going into the Marine Corps. But more importantly, my body and spirit were sending signals that this wasn't the right path for me and my health.

I was in Officer Candidate School (OCS), a nonstop ten-week boot camp for officers. OCS included intense physical, mental, academic, and leadership training.

During the program, they lined us up for required vaccinations. In hindsight, it took me years to realize that I was never the same after those shots. I went through the rest of training with a tight, clenched jaw, and experienced other ailments, including gastrointestinal issues, a hacking cough, fatigue, and depression. I felt like something had changed mentally. I didn't think much of those problems at the time. The regimented structure of OCS doesn't leave you time to think. I chalked up my symptoms to lack of sleep and overtraining and just pushed through as I have always done in the past. I never felt like the vaccine made me sick, although like half of my fellow candidates, I had a weird, uncontrollable, persistent cough for a week straight. I never felt fully the same afterwards.

Years later, when I began to untangle all the factors of my failing health that had brought me to the brink of death, I did some research on vaccines and learned that they can cause numerous side effects that are listed directly in the package inserts. These vaccines are loaded with poisons and toxins. I also learned that getting several shots all at once intramuscularly is not natural to the immune system and is not something that would ever happen in nature. I suspect that this onslaught of vaccines had a major part to play in my health struggles.

After spending every night of the OCS program meditating on whether I should stay or leave, I decided the Marine Corps wasn't my path. I made the tough and scary decision to decline my commission; I wasn't going to become a Marine Corps officer. Although they gave me an option to accept my commission within a year, I didn't change my mind. Instead, I went back home to New York.

I had no idea what I wanted to do—there was no way I was going to take a desk job ever again. My girlfriend's sister suggested I'd be a great trainer. I'd been in fitness my whole life, I realized, and I was a pretty good athlete, excelling at almost every sport. I could picture myself doing great as a trainer and loving work in a physical environment.

My career took off, and in a short amount of time I became

one of the most productive trainers nationwide at Equinox, the most competitive personal training company at the time. I then was promoted to fitness manager, overseeing sometimes forty trainers at a time. Shortly after, I was pursued to run personal training departments as a personal training manager at Crunch Fitness.

On top of the grind and stress of my work at the gym, I was picked to write training programs and do audio recordings and photo shoots for *Men's Health Magazine*. I was working out hard, and I had reached amazing levels of fitness and knowledge, and they wanted me to share that in the magazine.

I thought I was in good shape after OCS, but now I had *way* more training, knowledge, and focus, and by this point had earned the highest-level strength and conditioning certification (the Certified Strength and Conditioning Specialist designation, or CSCS, one of the only certifications that carries the clout of being put after PhD). I was physically and mentally the strongest I had ever been. But the truth was, I hadn't learned what *true* health was, and I was about to get the hardest lesson of my life.

I wasn't giving myself time to relax and recover from my intense training regimen. I was eating quick meals that I grabbed on the go, including pizza and pasta from conventional grains that were loaded with pesticides. This diet not only didn't agree with me, but it deprived my body of the crucial nutrients it needed to keep up with my stressful schedule. On top of these problems, my body was overloaded with toxins from previous manual labor jobs, medications I'd taken, and other environmental factors. I didn't know

I had a finite amount of energy. I was young and thought I was invincible. Life always has a way of setting us straight.

And as if all that weren't enough during this time, I also started training for a grueling race: The *Men's Health* Urbanathlon.

RUNNING INTO THE GROUND

The Urbanathlon was an eight-mile obstacle course from the upper west side of Manhattan down to Battery Park with various challenges along the way—things like jumping over New York City cabs and running up and down fifty flights of stairs. My goal was to win this race. My ego was involved since I'd written Urbanathlon-specific training programs that were featured in *Men's Health*.

Some days, I would work twelve or thirteen hours, and then go train, *hard*, with what little fuel I had in the tank. There was a building down the street from where I worked where I would go to run up the flights of stairs, and one day in the middle of my sprints up the stairs, I started to feel heaviness in my chest. From there, my performance just kept getting worse and worse. The more I pushed through, the more fatigued and run down my body became.

About two weeks before the race, I developed a cough, and I was incredibly fatigued. I stopped training. I couldn't figure out what was going wrong. I knew I had to give my body a rest, but I still had a commitment to the race. I had trained so hard for the race and wasn't ready to give it up. Giving up wasn't an option with my mindset.

The day of the race, I wasn't feeling better, but I refused to drop out. As I ran the course, my heart rate crept way above normal: typically, I could sprint for a mile and my heart rate wouldn't get above 193. During the race, it hit 204, which for me was a bad sign. I'd never seen my heart rate stay so high for so long.

Despite alarm bells going off in my head, I kept running and finished the race. In fact, I still finished in the top ten percent, only running at about fifty percent of my capacity. This result was frustrating because I knew that if I'd been healthy, I most likely would have won first place, which would have been a powerful testimony to my programs in *Men's Health*. My ego was too involved.

The race had wrecked me. The fatigue and respiratory issues I had been feeling eventually turned into walking pneumonia after the race. I was given prescriptions for antibiotics and steroids (both oral forms and inhalers). I would come to find out later how dangerous these antibiotics can be, and that they were potentially a major catalyst in my health crisis and chronic fatigue.

After I took these meds, my health spiraled downwards and never improved. Something was really wrong, but I had no idea what to do and how to fix it.

My buddy Miguel Bethelery, a healer with a PhD in molecular medicine, told me in an interview, "The pharmaceutical industry doesn't know how to help the body; that's not its job. As a scientist, when I worked in the pharmaceutical industry, the strategy was to inhibit things—it was to block the action of specific proteins and enzymes. When you block a protein, you block the body."[3]

Medication should only be used in dire situations. Many conditions can be healed naturally to a certain degree, and medication often impedes the healing process and can poison systems in the body. It doesn't allow the body to do what it's naturally designed to do. Nature provides the solutions.

But I didn't learn any of that until later. At that time in my life, despite having been so fit, I was out of touch with my body. At that point I knew how to get myself and others super fit, but I had no idea how to help my body heal itself and be truly healthy in mind, body and spirit.

PRESCRIPTION FOR DESTRUCTION

The word "antibiotic" means "against life." It's designed to kill bacteria throughout our bodies. An antibiotic is essentially an atom bomb in your gut. It indiscriminately kills cells throughout the body, even immune cells, neurons, bacterial cells, and tumor cells.

During my illness, I took Avelox, a fluoroquinolone, which is a group of antibiotics that are widely used despite documented, long-lasting side effects, including neurological issues, tendinopathy, muscle weakness, immune issues, exhaustion, loss of energy, muscle wasting,[4] anemia, neu-

---

3 Miguel Bethelery, in conversation with the author, January 10, 2019.

4 R. J. Williams, et al, "The Effect of Ciprofloxacin on Tendon, Paratenon, and Capsular Fibroblast Metabolism," *American Journal of Sports Medicine*, May 2000, 28(3): 364-9.

ropathy,[5] and brain fog just to name a few. For some patients, these complications continue years after taking a standard course of these medications and many people never make the connection between antibiotic use and their health issues.[6]

I am lucky I did. Fluoroquinolones are such powerful medications that using these drugs is like taking a small dose of chemotherapy.[7] Certain antibiotics have even been studied for use in treating bladder cancer.[8] You can find articles claiming that fluoroquinolones have an excellent safety record; but the problem is, those articles don't describe the effects these drugs have on cell mitochondria, which are the "powerhouses" of each of your cells. Mitochondria are responsible for energy production, so keeping your mitochondria healthy should be top on your list. Fluoroquinolones can destroy the mitochondria that provide energy in cells,[9] disrupt the mitochondrial DNA replication process, and cause oxidative stress and eventual cell death, resulting in long-lasting health issues for the patients who take them.[10]

What's more, we have a tolerance and toxicity threshold with

5   J. S. Cohen, "Peripheral Neuropathy Associated with Fluoroquinolones," *Annals of Pharmacotherapy*, December 2001, 35(12): 1540-7.

6   Beatrice Alexandra Golomb, Hayley Jean Koslik, and Alan J. Redd, "Fluoroquinolone-Induced Serious, Persistent, Multi-Symptom Adverse Effects," *BMJ Case Reports*, October 5, 2015.

7   Lisa Bloomquist, "Cipro, Levaquin and Avelox Are Chemo Drugs," *Hormones Matter*, April 28, 2014.

8   A. M. Kamat, J. I. DeHaven, and D. L. Lamm, "Quinolone Antibiotics: A Potential Adjunct to Intravesical Chemotherapy for Bladder Cancer," *Urology*, July 1999, 54(1): 56-61.

9   John Neustadt and Steve R. Pieczenik, "Medication-Induced Mitochondrial Damage and Disease," *Molecular Nutrition & Food Research*, 2008, 52: 780-788.

10 Krzysztof Michalak, et al, "Treatment of the Fluoroquinolone-Associated Disability: The Pathobiochemical Implications," *Oxidative Medicine and Cellular Longevity*, September 25, 2017.

these drugs,[11] meaning that the first prescription of an antibiotic may not create noticeable, detrimental complications, but the effects compound over subsequent doses. Your doctor will probably never tell you about these "black box" warnings. I believe I had a delayed reaction to the antibiotics I took, and that they created the severe issues that I grappled with for years afterward.

AVOIDING FLUOROQUINOLONES

Fluoroquinolone antibiotics are commonly prescribed for a variety of illnesses, but I can tell you as a person whose health was destroyed by these drugs that they should only be taken if your life is in serious danger. Fluoroquinolones include:

- Ciprofloxacin (Cipro)
- Levofloxacin (Levaquin/Quixin)
- Gatifloxacin (Tequin)
- Moxifloxacin (Avelox)
- Ofloxacin (Ocuflox/Floxin/Floxacin)
- Norfloxacin (Noroxin)
- Delafloxacin
- Gemifloxacin

The truth is, these drugs are poison to your mitochondria and your cells and should never be used except in last-resort situations.

---

11   Peter Karran, "Mechanisms of Tolerance to DNA Damaging Therapeutic Drugs," *Carcinogenesis*, December 2001, 22(12): 1931-7.

While I was on Avelox, after I took each pill, I would crash and instantly fall asleep. It's as if my system needed to shut down for a while. This developed into a pattern that became commonplace in my life for years to come. My girlfriend would take pictures of all the strange places and positions I would fall asleep in. There's one of me passed out on a couch in the center of a mall in Atlanta where we had been shopping together.

Even after the course of prescriptions was done, I continued to feel worse. Within months of finishing the race my mind and body physically changed for the worse in a drastic way. I *looked* terrible. My face had changed. My skin turned yellowish-brown from jaundice. I started to gain fat, and I lost all my muscle. I had serious gut problems. Before I got sick, went from looking like a professional athlete to looking like death. People were repelled by me.

I had signs of brain dysfunction, too, similar to dementia or autism. I put milk back into the kitchen cabinets instead of the fridge. I couldn't answer emails; I literally couldn't read them. I'd always been mildly dyslexic, but at that point I couldn't make sense of words at all, my ability to spell got way worse, my speech started changing, I couldn't remember numbers and I would constantly switch them around.

My personality changed. I had a hard time holding eye contact with people. It was like I knew the person who I truly was inside, but my true self was not showing up in reality. I had lost connection and my mind had become more juvenile; my thoughts were uncoordinated and underdeveloped. For over a year, I had an intense headache that felt like I was getting stabbed in the brainstem.

I later learned that these are all signs of gut dysfunction, which can cause extreme brain inflammation and neurological damage known as encephalopathy or encephalitis. Gut dysfunction can destroy the blood-brain barrier (BBB), which is a protective layer that defends the brain against pathogens, unwanted immune cells, heavy metals, cytokines, and other toxins. Think of the BBB as a thin protective paper film: when we are stressed from lack of sleep, WIFI exposure, or high blood pressure for example, these stressors create leaks in the BBB, like dabbing a lit cigarette to the paper film. Many of the techniques provided in this book will also help in one way or another to improve the integrity of the BBB.

The heaviness in my chest continued, and for a year or so it felt like someone was pressing down on it all the time. I couldn't breathe fully. I couldn't sleep properly, either. I'd get up at night with weird sensations of nervousness and anxiety, and I couldn't pinpoint why.

I went to a few different doctors during this time, but every one of them was stumped and kept saying the same thing: "I need to get a blood test." To address the gut pain I was experiencing, I drove to Savannah to see a gastroenterologist, who ordered yet another blood test.

The nurse, upon seeing my lab results, said, "Oh my God, your numbers are so great. I wish I had your blood."

I feel like absolute shit, I thought. *I'm in the worst condition of my entire life.* I've never felt worse than when I was told that my blood was perfect.

I began to doubt that conventional medicine held the answers for me. If a nurse was telling me things looked perfect when, clearly, everything was not perfect, then clearly something was missing.

Through a mastermind group, I'd met Peter Osbourne (the chiropractor I would later end up calling in the line at the pharmacy). Peter was known as the "gluten guy" for a book he'd written, *No Grain, No Pain*,[12] about the harm gluten creates for the gut. I described my symptoms to him during one of our mastermind meetings, and he suspected I was gluten intolerant. He gave me a few tips to try right away—the first one being to cut out gluten. Within just a few weeks of following his advice, I felt better than any of the interventions I'd gotten in hospitals and doctors' offices up to that point. My digestion improved, and I had less fatigue and mental fogginess. I was still sick, but there was clear improvement on some of my symptoms.

By this point, I was about a year into starting my own fitness center, and my girlfriend (now wife) and I lived in a loft above it—which meant I literally lived at work. This was probably not a good environment for healing, as I learned. The business was so demanding, and my condition had deteriorated so much, that I would just sleep and work, sleep and work. It was a struggle to live, let alone run a physically demanding business.

All these symptoms—the neurological issues, gastrointestinal distress and changes to my skin and physique—were layered over one another like a Jackson Pollock painting. The issues were complex and interdependent. Up close, each problem

---

12   Peter Osborne, *No Grain, No Pain*, New York: Atria Books, 2016.

was a single splatter of paint, but you had to step back to see the whole picture.

Health works this way for everyone. Everything is connected; no one body part functions separately. When we get ill, it doesn't happen overnight. Our bodies are miraculous. They're constantly working to heal us from the stressors we're exposed to. Those stressors layer over each other. If we're eating poorly and exposed to too many stressors, toxins, and chemicals and the body can't process it all, one of those stressors will become the last straw on the camel's back. Those toxic substances get stored in the organs, the joints, and the brain. They invade our systems and cause disease. The illness that results usually isn't the result of the single stressor that tipped the scales. It's an expression of all the underlying processes in our bodies that are overloaded. With the overload, we can fry our biological battery.

One day, about two years after the race, the scales finally tipped. I felt a searing, excruciating pain in my gut, and I dropped to the ground. On a scale from one to ten, this pain was a twelve. My girlfriend found me curled in a ball on the floor.

"Are you okay?" she asked.

"I don't know," was my honest answer. I had a very, very high tolerance for pain. I was used to pushing the limits of my mind and my body. But this was a pain unlike any I'd ever felt. Ask anyone who has had an intestinal blockage and they will all say it's an indescribably painful experience.

My girlfriend knew my pain tolerance. "I think we need to go to the hospital," she said.

At first, despite my reported pain levels at the hospital, the nurse thought it was just gastroenteritis, the technical term for a stomach bug. I said, "Have you ever had gastroenteritis? And you were in this much pain?" The nurse then told me I needed to go home and relax. I didn't believe I had gastroenteritis—I know what a stomach bug feels like, and this wasn't it—but she insisted. They had just discharged me when luckily an infectious disease doctor happened to take a look at my X-rays and scans. A nurse came running toward me as I was walking out the hospital doors.

"Hold up, hold up," she said, "we need you in here now."

By the grace of God or whatever higher power in the universe was watching over me, the doctor had noticed a twist or blockage on the scans and had told the staff I needed to be admitted immediately. The next thing I knew, I was on a gurney with tubes connected everywhere. I had a tube down my throat to my stomach, and my arms were stuck with IVs. I was given morphine. The pain was so intense that the morphine did absolutely nothing for me—if anything, it made me feel sicker. After about forty-eight hours of no sleeping and constant pain, they gave me Dilaudid, the strongest painkiller available.

There was a point during this ordeal where I didn't want to live anymore. *If it's going to be like this,* I thought, *I don't want to be part of it.* I was done with the pain and confusion; it was too much for too long. As the doctors performed test after test, they concluded I was very close to dying. If they didn't see signs of recovery soon, they were considering surgery to cut out the part of my intestine that was twisted and blocked.

After two days of pain, I finally passed out. And while it was a Dilaudid-induced sleep, it was the first opportunity for my body to start to heal. My intestine started to slowly turn back—which meant no surgery.

The next morning, I was brought a hospital breakfast consisting of coffee, Jell-O, pancakes, and bacon. I couldn't think of a worse meal for someone with gut trauma. I knew enough at the time to understand that the food I was being given would only make my situation worse. It was another "aha" moment: I realized that the medical system is not designed to heal, and doctors know nothing about nutrition. Food can be medicine or poison, and the hospital "nutritionist" was like a robot spewing out advice and knew nothing about the role of food in healing or health.

A quote from Winston Churchill came to mind: *If you're going through hell, keep going.*

I made a pact on that hospital bed: I wasn't going to give up and let go. I was going to get better. I was going to heal myself, one way or another and use it to inspire others who may be in a similar situation.

Every doctor had the same questions, the same process, and no solution. They looked at the Jackson Pollock mess of my disease one paint splatter at a time, and they kept shifting the diagnosis.

I had already been diagnosed with Lyme disease, and the last doctor at the hospital told me I also had Crohn's disease. "You can't cure it," he said, and he gave me the $1,800-per-month prescription that was basically a roll of the dice in terms of whether it would help. I thought, *This isn't a solution. This is on par with a placebo.*

I was at a crossroads. In the back of my mind, a nagging fear said, *You need to stop trying to control things. Just surrender to what they're telling you to do.* A friend of mine came in to visit me and said the same thing. Just do what they are telling you.

But a deeper intuition answered, *Something's not right here.*

That's how I found myself, in the prescription line at CVS, crying and emotional and utterly torn. I called my friend Peter, the "gluten guy."

That was the end of it for me. I was done with mainstream medicine.

PRESCRIPTION FOR HOPE

Through the same mastermind where I'd been introduced to Peter, another member told me about a healer in Hong Kong, David Jack, who helped heal a guy who had a strange brain fungus that no doctors had been able to figure out. I contacted him, and he sent me paperwork to fill out alongside instructions to mail him a sample of my hair.

He had me fill out a survey about emotional traumas, toxicity issues, and other illnesses in my medical history. *Did I have amalgam fillings in my teeth? What traumas had I had?* I told him about my recent hospitalization and my Crohn's diagnosis. I'd also been taking various cycles of antibiotics for the Lyme disease, and I'd been on doxycycline and amoxicillin consistently over the past eight months.

"You can continue to take the antibiotics if you want," David Jack said when we got on the phone for a consultation, "but you don't need to."

This was news to me—every medical professional I'd encountered had told me it's important to finish a cycle of antibiotics once you've begun it. But David Jack asserted that my body could heal on its own. I decided to trust him. I stopped taking the meds, and I started his holistic protocol instead.

With his guidance, I started to prepare for a heavy-metal detox, and started to naturally kill off the microbes living in my gut. Within three months, David Jack got me feeling better than any doctor had before (in fact, every other conventional doctor had made me feel worse in the end). He first had me remove my amalgam fillings, which had been leaching heavy metals into my body since I was a kid—and this, it turned out, was a big piece of my health problem. I'd had a stabbing pain in the back of my head that dramatically reduced as soon as I got my amalgam fillings out (we'll look at amalgam fillings and other toxins in more depth in chapter six).

David Jack had me take core minerals and vitamins I'd been deficient in. After I started taking them, I felt like I could feel the toxins and heavy metals start to process out of my brain. David Jack started me on the right path, but it was really only the beginning because little did I know I was so far down the rabbit hole of ill health it was going to take years and most of my excess time, money, and energy to find some semblance of normalcy.

SEEKING TRUTH IN NATURE

I began to research a wide variety of holistic healers and natural healing protocols, and I realized that there is a lot of conflicting advice between conventional medicine and holistic approaches. It was difficult to tease out the best healing path. But because I had been on the brink of death, I was willing to try anything. I had already tried what Western medicine had to offer, and Chinese medicine gave me a glimpse of hope. I began to experiment with all the healing practices I came across to understand what would work for me.

Through all my research, I was beginning to see health from a new perspective. In our modern Western culture, we've been taught that we need medical intervention to care for ourselves, and that our bodies will not heal on their own and we must depend on doctors. We take medications to block specific symptoms, but the root cause of disease goes unaddressed. In the long run, many times the medication complicates the situation or makes everything worse.

But what if we instead focus on supporting our body's own natural healing systems? To look at health holistically, through the lens of what the body needs (instead of what symptom needs to be fixed), we have to reconnect to ourselves, and bring our body back to nature. *We are nature.* Everything is connected and affected by another part of the body. Nothing works in isolation like doctors will have you believe.

This concept was at first unfamiliar to me. As a competitive athlete, I had been taught to ignore my body's complaints and push through them. For example, as young as six years old, I started competing at a high level in swimming, and at ten years old, I entered a competition for a five-mile swim in a lake. I had very low body fat, I was thin and had to be pulled out about two and a half miles in because my lips turned purple and I began to get hypothermic. By the time I was ten, I had broken both collar bones and both arms through various feats.

To make it through OCS for the Marine Corps, you have to just numb out and push through discomfort and pain. This was the norm. This was something I was used to doing my whole life. I had to ignore the fatigue and gastrointestinal distress I was experiencing in order to get the job done.

That's what so many of us do—we dissociate and disconnect from our bodies. As a result, we miss the signs and symptoms that our bodies are telling us about what is wrong and how to heal.

To understand your body's natural processes, Miguel Bethelery says to consider how a baby operates. When a baby is born, the first thing they do is breathe. The word "inspiration" actually means, "to breathe in"—at the most basic level, breathing connects us to the source of life. "Breathing is our first food." Bethelery says it is the most important nutrient, "and that's why breathwork is so powerful. You can do a lot with breathwork, and only with that."[13] Observe sometime how a baby naturally breathes: they breathe in through the nose and their belly expands.

This is the first step in observing your own state. Simply

---

13   Miguel Bethelery, in conversation with the author, January 10, 2019.

look at how you're breathing. Do you breathe into your chest all day? Do you breathe in through your mouth? Are your breaths constantly shallow? Are you breathing heavily? Do you constantly hold tension in some part of your body? All of these changes in the breath signal that your body is stressed.

Our breathing becomes more rapid and shallow when we're stressed and in "fight or flight" mode. In fight or flight, the body engages all the systems that help us survive, and it shuts down the systems that help us heal and recover.

If you're living in that state all day every day, the body will burn out. In fight or flight, cortisol levels stay up and adrenal fatigue can set in depending on the strength of the organism. Oxygen is essential to healing, alongside carbon dioxide, as you will see later.

The second thing a baby does is feed, and they're put to their mother's breast. "The baby is going to be eating the food that's most appropriate for them," Bethelery says, and it's equally important for us to continue to eat what's most appropriate for us as we grow. Look to the source of your food. Are you feeding your body what it needs? Are you eating processed foods, or real nutrition from the breast of Mother Earth—fruits, vegetables, and lean meats? Our diet gives our bodies the vitamins, minerals, and essential nutrients we need to function.

The third thing a baby does is eliminate. "You need to be able to eliminate the residues of your digestion," Bethelery says, "but you also need to eliminate poisons, you need to eliminate toxins, and you need to eliminate things that are not needed or wanted by your body." Look to your own bowel movements for signs of distress. Are you constipated or going to the bathroom frequently? Is your stool liquid and loose, or nice and firm? Is there mucus? Do you leave skid marks in the toilet? These are all signs there may be an issue. The quality of your bowel movements can tell you a lot about your body's overall health.

The last thing a baby does is sleep. What are your sleep patterns like? Are you consistently going into a deep sleep, or are you waking constantly throughout the night? Do you feel fully rested when you wake up, or do you feel like you could sleep for another three hours? Most of our body's recovery processes take place while we're sleeping. Poor sleep results in poor recovery. One thing is for sure, you will never heal if you can't consistently go into deep recovery sleep.

Compare the natural behaviors of a baby to the way many people operate in modern life: modern adults wake up late after hitting their alarm a bunch of times, rush around to get ready for the day, and grab a cup of coffee. They hop in their car and get stressed out in traffic. On the news piped in from the radio, they're bombarded with tons of fear-based information that fires up their reptilian survivalist brain (which has also been activated and accelerated by that cup of coffee). They run into work, to a job they likely hate. They get run down at their job all day and are typically eating junk, and then they get back in their car, drive home in traffic, and have a couple of drinks to unwind before they go to bed. The alcohol screws up their sleep, and they don't go into deep REM sleep. The next morning, not fully rested, they wake up again to the alarm that they snooze, hoping for a little more rest.

These four elements—breathing, eating, eliminating, and

sleeping—can indicate a person's total health. If one of those elements is off, you won't be performing at your optimal levels. If two of those elements are off, disease and discomfort set in. When three of those elements are out of alignment, you're most likely in serious trouble. By noticing how you're doing with these basics, you can bring dis-ease back to health.

BASIC HEALTH SELF-ASSESSMENT

When I work with clients, I have them fill out a simple self-assessment to determine their current state of health and the level they want to get to. Grab a pen and paper and write down your thoughts on the following:

Where Are You Now? On a scale from one (poor) to ten (perfect), use your intuition to rate how you're doing with:
- Breathing patterns
- Digestion and elimination
- Uninterrupted sleep
- Clean water intake
- Clean Fruit intake
- Clean Veggie intake
- Daily exercise
- Daily time spent outdoors in the sun or connected to nature

Where Do You Want to Go? For each of the above categories, write down the rating you want to achieve.

Why Do You Want This? Write down all the reasons that motivate you to improve your health. Visualize how you want to feel. At what level do you want to perform? By this time next year, what needs to happen for you to feel happy about your results?

How Are You Going to Get There? Write down your plan to improve your habits in each of the above categories and focus on one thing at a time. As you read this book and learn the hacks that influence the health of specific systems of your body, return to this plan to modify and add to it. If you can envision and prepare in the mind's eye where you want to be, you are close to making that outcome a reality. If daily exercise is really low, then focus on doing one to five minutes a day in your first week and go from there.

As I continued on my healing journey, I realized that I needed to define for myself what health and healing really meant. David Jack had given me detox and healing protocols to follow; after I'd completed them, I felt better and he said I was completely healed. But that wasn't the end. I knew I had further to go—the only benchmark I had to compare myself to was the high level of performance I'd reached before I'd gotten sick. What did it really mean to me to be healthy?

Miguel Bethelery says, "Healing isn't a mind thing—it's the process of the mind learning to step away from what the body needs to do."[14] For me, healing is coming back to nature and being in harmony. And in the next chapter, we'll take a look at what that means.

---

14   Miguel Bethelery, in conversation with the author, January 10, 2019.

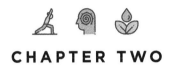

CHAPTER TWO

HOW THOUGHTS BECOME ACTION

David Hawkins, the nationally-renowned psychiatrist, physician, researcher, spiritual teacher, and lecturer, proposed that everything in the universe—including our thoughts and feelings—operates on a scale of consciousness. Hawkins classified consciousness, including thoughts and feelings, into a scale that can be measured, from low-vibration thoughts, such as shame, to high-vibration thoughts, such as love.

This philosophy connected many of the dots for me. As Hawkins describes it:

> The "Map of Consciousness" illuminates unknown aspects of consciousness. With each progressive rise in the level of consciousness, the "frequency" or "vibration" of energy increases. Thus, higher consciousness radiates a beneficial and healing effect on the world, verifiable in the human muscle response which stays strong in the presence of love and truth. In contrast, non-true or negative energy fields which "calibrate" below the level of integrity induce a weak-muscle response. This stunning discovery of the difference

between "power" and "force" has influenced numerous fields of human endeavor: business, advertising, education, psychology, medicine, law, and international relations.[15]

One of the most powerful and factual ways to understand this is the placebo effect: When you take a sugar pill and have a belief that it is healing you, it is actually the belief alone that heals you. Your perception of the healing that was occurring created emotions and thoughts, and those emotions and thoughts created the chemicals your body needs to heal itself. So, your thoughts and beliefs are the supplement and the medication.

We are the only species that can create our own environment. It is a gift. We have the human brain, which allows us to create through our words, thoughts, feelings, and actions. We manifest our reality based on those things and our perception affects each one of them. When we take inventory of our thoughts, feelings and actions, and we begin to see how life has unfolded and manifested as a result, we can start to take responsibility for where we are, and there is a saying I love, which I picked up from a good friend: "If I am not the problem, then there is no solution." I assume you want a solution, right? Much of the time, that's where healing begins.

As I began to do personal inventory with questions like, *Why am I here?* and, *What is my purpose?* I came to understand that my sole purpose is to help people raise their consciousness, frequency, and vibration, heal their bodies and minds, and feel the *true* freedom that comes with it—as I have experienced.

---

15   "Dr. Hawkins Biography," *Veritas Publishing*, 2017.

Maya Angelou said, "Success is liking yourself." "Success" can be replaced with "healing," and" liking" with "love." Healing is loving yourself.

In what parts of your life do you have patterns of resentment, blame, shame, guilt, anger, and frustration? On the flip side of that, where and how could you break those patterns and create more forgiveness, love, peace, and happiness?

When we're not in alignment with our higher selves, we become disconnected from our true being.

THE ROOT CAUSE OF DIS-EASE

Through my own personal experience, my ten years of research into healing, and the work of the many healers I've learned from, I've come to understand that the root cause of dis-ease is our disconnection with ourselves and with nature. We are part of nature, so disconnecting from nature is disconnection from self. Often, this disconnection can begin as a result of physical or emotional trauma.

When a person experiences trauma, it can create a disconnect from the true self and affect their belief system. If someone was told repeatedly the idea that they were worthless at a young age (or if this idea was literally beaten into them), they may take that belief, thought and feeling with them. When someone believes they're worthless, they may do destructive things to their body. They might use drinking to numb themselves from the pain and trauma, for example. They will become more disconnected from their body's signs of health, and more vulnerable to disease.

The pain created by trauma, if not addressed, can and often does lead to some form of addiction as the person tries to push the pain away rather than confronting or dealing with it. They might become emotional over-eaters or workaholics; they might exercise themselves to death or just look at their phone all day to disassociate and not feel.

Gabor Maté, the renowned physician with a focus on child development and trauma, says, "Don't ask the question, 'Why the addiction?' but 'Why the pain?' Addiction is only a symptom; it's not the fundamental problem. The fundamental problem is trauma." The first step in healing is understanding what we are disconnecting from.

It's typical for people in general in our society but even more so for those who had traumatic childhoods, that we disconnect from our true nature and true being, which is pure love, joy, and happiness. As we disconnect, we also numb our biofeedback mechanisms. We don't feel our body's indicators that tell us something is wrong. Instead, we push through and stuff feelings deep down until our body's signals get loud enough to hear. Pain is a great teacher. The body is a great feedback mechanism.

Biomed technician and engineer John McMullin studies how our perceptions affect our energy and our physiology. "Trauma is what puts you to sleep," he says, "and trauma is what wakes you up."[16] We can begin to heal when we take responsibility for the actions that have brought us dis-ease. When we understand the beliefs that are at the root of our actions, we can begin to shift.

---

16 John McMullin, in conversation with the author, June 4, 2019.

HOW WE CREATE BELIEFS

The words we use carry specific feelings and even vibrations with them. Each word we speak has a vibration that is rooted in truth or removed from truth. I illustrate this to my coaching groups with a simple exercise: first, I have them repeat, "I should, I want, I could, and I am going to," over and over for a minute or so, and then I ask them to check in with how they feel in their body.

Then, I ask the group to repeat, "I am," and "I do," over and over for another minute or so. When I ask them to check in with how they feel, they notice a difference in quality between the first and second set.

The first set of phrases are about the past or the future; they're disconnected from the current reality. Think of what emotions come up when someone says to us, we "should" do something—typically, we get inflamed. "Should" carries judgment, and we can feel the irritation that arises from that judgment in our bodies. A victim mindset is typically stuck in the past.

But the second set of phrases are rooted in the present moment. The present-moment phrases are resonating in the truth, because there is no other time than the present. When we speak in the now, we're connected to the truth of what is.

However, we are frequently pulled out of the here and now by the stories we construct as we worry about the future or remember distressing events from the past. Our beliefs result from these stories, which become powerful tools for shaping our reality. Our ego may inject itself when remembering what happened and tell the story in a different way because of how we view the world.

For example, if a person's parents got divorced when they were young, and their dad left, that person may have a story of victimhood that comes from a belief that they are not loved or that men are abandoners. The person then looks for validation of their story. This idea that they are unloved may be an unconscious one based on a single event or multiple instances, but that story produces thoughts, which create feelings, which ultimately produce action in the world. This person may walk around with deep anger and resentment that get stored in the emotional centers of the brain blocking this person from being the best version of himself.

These complex stories of the self become our ego, which exists to protect us and help us relate to the world. Our life experiences, particularly those that happen at a young age, shape our view of the world. We may search for evidence to reinforce those views, and if we find enough evidence to confirm our story, we can create an ingrained belief that is not necessarily true.

This can have massive effects on the rest of our lives. If we believe X, than all opposition to X is usually threatening to our ego. The ego is tricky: it can prevent us from taking responsibility for our lives, causing us to blame others and frame ourselves as victims. This can close off opportunities, restrict possibilities, and prevent people from entering your life. The ego can be extremely damaging.

Many of our core beliefs are set by the time we're seven years old. Before age seven, our brains operate at a lower frequency, dominated by theta brainwaves, which is similar to a hypnotic state where the subconscious is susceptible to programming.[17] As the brain matures around age seven, the experiences and programming that came before that point tend to become more set. From that point on, we're running the program from earlier years. We are all basically little kids pretending to be mature adults.

An example of this is how people's belief systems around money are formed. Many people's ideas of money are rooted in their parents' belief systems that they heard over and over again at a young age. Maybe they heard, "We don't have enough money," "You think I am made of money," "You've got to work hard for your money," "Money is the root of all evil," "Rich people are the problem," or "Money doesn't grow on trees." Whatever that message was, it formed the programming and associations that person has around money as they grow up.

The same goes for health. I can't tell you how many people that I see who are yo-yo dieters and have serious weight problems, and when I ask about their childhood, they describe how their parents put a huge emphasis on eating a certain way or shamed them for gaining weight.

These belief systems affect our health, but more importantly, they affect our self-worth. In an interview with me, John McMullin described how traumatic emotional experiences can create irritations and injuries in our physical bodies. McMullin looks at the language and metaphors we use to describe our feelings: our shoulders are "carrying the weight of the world," or someone "breaks" our heart. We use these metaphors because our bodies experience symptoms of

17   Bruce Lipton, "Are You Programmed at Birth?" *Heal Your Life*, August 17, 2010.

our emotional states. "Learning the language of the metaphoric discussion with the heart creates a new frequency and an opportunity," he said. By looking at the underlying emotional issue, we have an opportunity to heal the whole system, instead of just addressing the physical symptom.[18] The language we use to speak to ourselves and others has the power to change our reality and our health.

Our body is constantly giving us signs about our health, and we may choose to ignore them based on our beliefs about ourselves. That's how it was for me. I remember thinking that things were coming to me too easily; I needed a real challenge in life. As the Urbanathlon came closer I said, *I would rather die than not run this race.*

And guess what? I almost died—and I encountered the biggest challenge I would and probably ever face in my life: getting my health back while running a business.

I was the creator of that. I chose not to honor my body. I believed I was invincible. I thought I was a machine, that I could push through anything and rebound as I had done in the past. I ran my body down, and I burned it out. In essence, we are electrical beings, "bio batteries" with the power to light up a major city for an entire night. But just like solar panels need recharging, so does the body.

If other people treated us the way we treat ourselves at times, we may react with violence and anger or at least run away from the disrespect and pain. Why don't we treat ourselves the way we expect others to treat us? If a person beat us

---

18   John McMullin, in conversation with the author, June 4, 2019.

up, we wouldn't hang around them—yet people beat themselves up every day. Disease can be created when we treat ourselves negatively and ignore our physical symptoms. We can become our own worst enemy. The good news is that we can also become our own biggest supporter.

Once I understood how my beliefs had influenced my lack of self-care, I could take full responsibility for how I became sick. I saw how my thoughts had created my reality. My behaviors were rooted in belief systems that didn't serve me, and I almost killed myself over them.

Ego, which helps keep us alive at times, can also form distorted programmed beliefs. The ego is designed to protect us from pain—but it can also block us from the truth. Ego develops to prevent not just our physical death, but the death of our identities, our social connections, and even our fantasies, illusions and beliefs. As John McMullin says, "Ego doesn't like getting information that it can't hide."[19] An unhealthy ego can disconnect us from the present, and it can even make it painful for us to face reality. Remember, our programmed stories impact our thoughts and feelings, and ultimately our actions.

Friedrich Nietzsche said, "Sometimes people don't want to hear the truth because they don't want their illusions destroyed." We manifest the reality of our ego, good or bad, and the ego is great at creating illusions.

---

19   John McMullin, in conversation with the author, June 4, 2019.

GOD | SPIRIT | UNIVERSE | SOURCE ENERGY

We are born with pure consciousness and no ego
We learn to walk, talk and relate to the world

THE EGO IS BORN

We may consciously or unconsciously find evidence that reinforce those views

Since subconscious programming and beliefs are generally created under the age of 7 we may not be aware of how our beliefs are affecting perception and reality

We have experiences which may shape our views of self and the world (may or may not be true)

With enough evidence or even without it we can create a belief/s

The ego creates stories and beliefs to help us relate to our experiences and desires and protect us from pain. (The truth can be painful.)

Those beliefs and stories impact every:

THOUGHT	FEELING	WORD	ACTION

These 4 Things Manifest Our Reality
Don't like your current situation or reality?

Consider transforming beliefs and stories that don't serve you

Are your actions and words coming from the ego or the spirit?

Create new stories and beliefs that elevate and transform your life

Consider inventorying your thoughts, feelings, sayings, beliefs and stories for lack of truth

Consider aligning every thought, word, feeling and action with truth

Consider framing old stories with more positivity/gratitude, find the silver lining.

CHOICES

EGO		VS	SPIRITUALITY	
• In-authentic self	• Fraud • Non-truth		• Authentic self	• Inspiration (In spirit, to breathe in)
• Materialistic	• Suffering • Lower Dimensions		• Passions	• Higher Calling/Dimension
• Disease	• Selfish (me, mine, I)		• TRUTH	• Real happiness, love, joy, peace
			• Healing	

When the pain from the EGO becomes too great, awakening/transformations may occur

Both paths can lead to elevated consciousness or awakening

I had to learn the hard way that my will can only take me so far. I had to learn the laws of nature again. I had disconnected from my spiritual practices, and in my quest to recover,

I remembered that healing is a spiritual game. "To inspire" means "in spirit," which comes from root words meaning "to breathe in." And that's one of the many ways I started to reconnect with myself—by taking in breath, slowing down, and meditating. I began to have different thoughts, feelings, and actions that were based in my higher self instead of my ego. I started to realize that each time I'd refused to listen to my higher self, I had created the pain and suffering I was now encountering.

SHAPING OUR STORIES

"Anger is an acid that can do more harm to the vessel in which it is stored than to anything on which it is poured."

—MARK TWAIN

In *Love Yourself Like Your Life Depends On It*, author Kamal Ravikant tells his own personal story of reshaping his thoughts. Ravikant hated his life and was plagued by thoughts of suicide. One day, he decided he would look at himself in the mirror each day and repeat, "I love myself. I love myself. I love myself." In the book, Ravikant describes how this practice got him out of his dark hole, and his life began to improve. Each time he had a negative thought, he would follow it by saying, "I love myself." His words had the power to reshape his outlook on life.[20]

I didn't know it at the time, but I had used this technique when I was in my early twenties, long before I became sick, to get myself out of a dark place. Each time negative thoughts came up, I would acknowledge the story I was telling myself,

---

20   Kamal Ravikant, *Love Yourself Like Your Life Depends On It*, Love Yourself, 2012.

and the emotions that story was rooted in, such as fear, shame, guilt, remorse, anger, and jealousy. I then told myself positive thoughts to counter any negative thought I had popping up in my head, and I repeated them over and over again. Over time, this practice rewired the patterns of my thoughts. I began to see the power, influence, and impact that thoughts and mantras can have on our reality. When I read this book later in my life, during the time when I was sick, it hit me again how people who are stuck in a negative story can create a reality through focused thoughts and words. It is a practice that is so successful that I use it with my clients. I should add that the practice of repeating mantras won't necessarily reprogram the brain, but it does help move in that direction—and it has helped me and many others. A specific mantra I used while healing comes from a great book called *The Power of Your Subconscious Mind*:[21]

> "My body and all its organs were created by the infinite intelligence in my subconscious mind. It knows how to heal me. Its wisdom fashioned all my organs, tissues, muscles, and bones. This infinite healing presence within me is now transforming every cell of my being, making me whole and perfect. I give thanks for the healing I know is taking place at this time. Wonderful are the works of the creative intelligence within me."

---

21 Joseph Murphy, *The Power of Your Subconscious Mind*, Eastford, CT: Martino Publishing, 2011.

INVENTORY YOUR STORIES

Throughout your day, observe the times that negative thoughts come to mind. Each time these thoughts pop up, write them down. You can use the following questions to help you take inventory:

- When was I fearful today?
- When was I dishonest?
- When was I angry or frustrated?
- When was I selfish?
- Do I owe anyone an apology?
- Did I gossip?
- Do I need to forgive someone?
- Was I defensive?
- Did I paint myself a victim?
- Did I gain any resentments?

(As a side note, the word "resentment" comes from the Latin words "re," meaning "again," and "sentere," meaning "to feel." Resentment, then, means to "re-feel." You can recognize resentment by how it makes you feel after an event has already passed. You are holding on to resentment if, for example, you still get angry when you think of a certain person. There is an old saying that goes, "Resentments are like drinking poison and hoping the other person will die.")

Next, take a moment to write down where these thoughts come from. What in your past shaped this line of thinking? What are the stories you're creating around these thoughts?

Then, consider what story would create a positive, healing shift around that thought. What is the inverse of that thought and how can you express it? What do you need to hear right now? How can you express love for yourself?

Our stories become beliefs through repetition. Our old, negative stories were reinforced by our past—but we can replace them with new, positive stories the more often we practice shifting our thinking. This practice only takes a moment and can create lasting, positive shifts in your thought patterns and your overall health and wellbeing.[22] There is also a saying that I love which is, "All positive thought is prayer." The inverse of that, as Michael Pritchard famously described it, is: "Fear is that little darkroom where negatives are developed."

OUR SELF-REGULATING SYSTEM

Amazing scientific studies have shown that your emotions affect your DNA.[23] In one experiment, DNA was taken from a subject and placed in a sealed tight container. Emotional stimuli was given to the DNA donor, and the results were fascinating: Positive emotions caused the DNA to relax, whereas negative emotions caused the DNA to constrict and tighten.

In another study, scientists concluded that our DNA shapes the behavior of light photons, which in turn make up our visible reality. The experimenters put light photons in a vacuum and observed them; then they inserted DNA into the vacuum, and the photons started following the geometry of the DNA.

---

22 Christian Jarrett, "The Transformational Power of How You Talk About Your Life," *BBC*, May 27, 2019.

23 Greg Braden, "DNA Report," *Electrical Inkblot Garden*, May 2005.

Lastly another study was done by taking white blood cells and putting them in a chamber to measure the electrical activity of the cells. The subject was placed in the room and provided emotional stimulation in the form of video clips. The DNA and the donor were monitored from their respective rooms, and as the emotional stimulus provided peaks and valleys, the electrical responses to both the DNA and the donor had the same response at the same time—even up to fifty miles away. This means that the donor and the DNA were connected beyond space and time.

In short, there is a link between our emotions the action of our DNA. If we accept that our DNA can alter our reality (which we'll talk about more in a moment), then that can only mean that our feelings and emotions are quite literally shaping the world around us. We are choosing our reality by the attitude that we carry around with us day by day. The world can only be a reflection of the feelings we hold in our bodies. HeartMath researchers have gone so far as to show that physical aspects of DNA strands could be influenced by human intention.[24]

When we feel stressed, there is a physiological cascade of events that takes place and can vary dramatically from person to person. This is due to many factors, including nature and nurture. Finding out how you handle and react to stress is important. Imagine, for example, that someone has a stressful day at work, and their coping mechanism or natural reaction is to instantly soothe the anxiety about everything they have to do, so they grab a fast-food meal and they eat it on the go. They don't hydrate because they're not paying

---

24 "You Can Change Your DNA," *HeartMath Institute*, July 14, 2011.

attention to their thirst. They don't stop to rest, digest, and calm down.

The body may be able to deal with a single day of this kind of neglect, but string a series of days or years together and dis-ease can arise. The time it takes to reach a breaking point all depends on the strength of the organism, among many other factors.

Yale psychologists McEwen and Stellar coined the term *allostatic load* in 1993 to describe the effects of the sum total of stressors that your body accumulates over time. The body is always trying to reach homeostasis, so in response to challenges (like a fast food meal on the go), a variety of processes cause fluctuations in endocrine and neural responses. When these challenges are repetitive and chronic, they cause wear and tear on the body.

This one stressful day creates a small problem for the body to solve. The fast-food meal is not only hard to process, devoid of nutrients and full of chemicals, but because the body isn't well hydrated, it struggles to clear waste products from the cells. The immune system may switch on if it feels the foreign substances need to be addressed, and this can lead to an overactive immune system. Inflammation may occur due to the stressful environment, negative emotions and the chemicals in the non-food food. Meanwhile, this person's blood pressure stays high all day long, trying to keep up with the demands of rushing from one thing to the next and not giving the body what it needs physically, mentally, and emotionally— which is some downtime and good nutrients.

These inflammatory and immune responses are part of our

self-regulating system; it's the body just trying to do its job. It's supposed to get inflamed as a natural part of healing and recovery, just as when you work out or sprain an ankle. In the case of an illness, the immune system kicks in to clean up pathogens, and tamps back down once the pathogens have been removed. But when the pathogens can't be identified, the immune system can start attacking parts of the body. We call this process autoimmune disease.

When our bodies are consistently dealing with stress—in the form of emotional trauma, negative behaviors, or even a toxic environment—our bodies become overwhelmed, and inflammatory issues start to rear their ugly heads. When we're continually stressed out and the immune system is trying to fend off invaders, that consistent, low-grade inflammation can become a major problem. In fact, all disease begins with inflammation. Not to mention, constant low-grade chronic inflammation can remove and destroy motivation by reducing dopamine in the brain.[25]

In autoimmune diseases, white blood cells don't just attack foreign invaders—they can end up attacking any tissues (including normal body tissues) that may mimic or look similar to toxins, foods, or other foreign particles. For some people, gluten molecules look similar to thyroid tissues; when the body is overloaded with gluten, it can attack the thyroid as well, resulting in Hashimoto's disease. Rheumatoid arthritis, for example, happens when the body attacks the joints. Crohn's disease—the condition I was diagnosed with—happens when the body is attacking part of the intestines.

---

25   Michael T. Treadway, Jessica A. Cooper, and Andrew H. Miller, "Can't or Won't? Immunometabolic Constraints on Dopaminergic Drive," *Trends in Cognitive Sciences*, April 1, 2019, 23(5): 435-448.

In an interview I did with pharmacologist Dr. TK Huynh, he defined healing as, "activating the body's system to be able to go back into homeostasis."[26] Our bodies are always trying to rebalance themselves and get back to physical homeostasis, but as Huynh describes, our conscious and unconscious mind can sometimes scramble the instructions for getting back to the body's normal state. "A lot of the time, trauma, emotional stress, physical stress, or pain can interfere with this homeostatic system," he said. "If we could easily use a very safe way, without synthetic drugs and harmful side effects, to instruct the body to get back to normal physically and emotionally—that would be the journey of healing." Our bodies work just like animals' bodies do in nature—they aren't given blood pressure meds or cholesterol meds to heal.

PICKING UP THE FREQUENCIES OF HEALING

To understand more fully how emotional stress becomes inflammation and physical disease, we have to understand how emotions trigger the nervous system.

When we're in states of stress, fear, anxiety, and anger, our bodies are in sympathetic arousal—the unconscious system that directs whether we fight, flee, or freeze in response to a threat. In this mode, our bodies are releasing adrenaline, releasing glucose from the liver, sending blood to the extremities, pumping cortisol (the stress hormone), and increasing inflammation to protect tissues. These feelings produce acids, which literally poison the body. When we experience joy, and peace, our system begins to relax, and the parasympathetic system kicks in. This is where rest, relaxation, digestion, and

---

26   Dr. TK Huynh, in conversation with the author, May 8, 2019.

recuperation happen. When we're in parasympathetic mode, our cortisol and inflammation levels go down.

Remember David Hawkins' work: thoughts and feelings on the lower half of the scale of consciousness are destructive to life and the cells—meaning they cause our energy to contract. In a state of contraction, no energy can flow, and they put us in a sympathetic fight-or-flight response. Thoughts and feelings on the upper half of the scale are constructive to life; they're experiences we're drawn toward, and they increase our ability to turn on the restorative parasympathetic system and allow "good vibes" to flow freely.

Bruce Lipton uses the metaphor of cellular antennae to illustrate how we can tap into higher-frequency experiences. Back in the days of a TV set with antennae, you could choose a channel and adjust the antennae to pick up a broadcast. The broadcast was always there, traveling as a frequency through space, and whether we picked up the program was a matter of which channel we chose and how we adjusted the conditions to receive it.

Similarly, Lipton says that all of our cells have antennae, and they pick up frequencies that either attract or repel us from particular stimuli and environments. Our body then creates movement, or action, based on the frequencies it picks up, which could come from food, other people, electrical appliances, or environmental fields.

An environment of fear causes constriction; we pull away from stimulus that is threatening. We pull away from something we are scared of, or we may even pull away from the best, most life-changing thing in the world because we are afraid to change.

An environment of love, gratitude, peace, and joy, on the other hand, allows us to expand. This is the environment that allows our system to thrive and our bodies to heal.

These environments affect us within and without: they influence our actions and behaviors, and within our bodies, they influence the way our cells react and the chemicals they produce. These chemicals affect our neurochemistry, our cellular processes, and our epigenetics, as our environment, both the internal environment of our bodies and external environment around us, can cause a switch to turn genes off or on. Just think of how different your action would be if you made decisions based on fear vs. love.

You don't need science to explain this; you don't even need to believe in the idea of frequency to feel how it operates in your body. You can see how this works with a short exercise: think of a time when you felt the most peace and love in your life. Hold that memory in your mind and visualize it in as much detail as you can. Let the feelings of that memory permeate every cell of your being.

Now place your hand over your heart and think of something you're deeply grateful for. Let those feelings of gratitude permeate every cell of your being. Feel the feeling of gratitude all over.

Notice how your body feels when you hold peace, love, and gratitude in your mind and heart. When we're truly connected with our gratitude and our feelings when we're in a high-vibration state of love, joy, and peace, we can feel the shift in our bodies. That sense of relaxation is a signal that the healing process has been stimulated in the parasympathetic nervous system.

Every time your heart pumps with gratitude, it sends that energy—just like a sonar pulse—out into the world. The world around you picks up that message, whether consciously or unconsciously. The responses you receive from the world are a direct reflection of those thoughts and feelings that you have carried with you and sent out into the world. In fact, right now, you are the sum total of all the thoughts, feelings, and actions that you have put out into the world—if that weren't true, you would be somewhere else. If you don't like your current situation, I have great news for you: you can change it in an instant.

If you want a particular type of tree to grow in your garden, you must deliberately choose the seeds you plant. How often do you care for your garden? Is it possible that the grass looks greener on the other side because it is getting more care? How often do you remove the weeds from your mind?

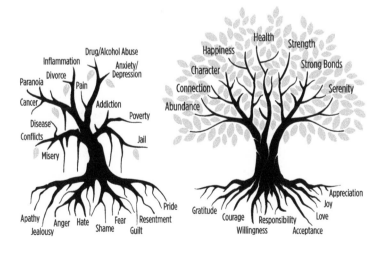

CHANGE YOUR THOUGHTS, CHANGE YOUR HEALTH

Many people are willing to work out to get six-pack abs, but few think about how to train their mental and emotional health. They rarely thing about a "six-pack heart."

The heart is constantly sending neurological information to the brain and the rest of the body. On a biochemical level, the heart releases atrial peptides that inhibit the release of stress hormones in the brain. Literal energy waves are sent out in the heart's pulse and blood pressure, and the electrical energy of our pulse creates measurable electrical surges in the brain, like sonar from a submarine. Not only can this pulse be measured from anywhere on our body, but it is broadcast into the environment around us, pulsed out into the world and out into the universe.

This interconnectivity becomes even more important when we consider that our emotions have a direct physical effect on the heart. Sandeep Jauhar is the director of the heart failure program at Long Island Jewish Medical Center, as well as a two-time bestselling author. He asserts that our emotions can change the heart's shape and structure. In a TEDx talk, he described the interactions between our emotions and our heart's response:

> Fear and grief can cause profound cardiac injury. The nerves that control the unconscious processes, such as the heartbeat, can sense distress and trigger a maladaptive fight-or-flight response. Blood vessels constrict, causing the heart to gallop and blood pressure to rise. In other words, it is clear that our hearts are extraordinarily sensitive to our emotions.[27]

---

27   Sandeep Jauhar, "How Your Emotions Change the Shape of Your Heart," *TED*, 2019.

So you are not just what you eat—you are also what you feel. What you put in your mouth is important, but even more important may be what you put into your heart and your mind about the thing you are eating. The energy you put out is a product of what you've watched, read, and surrounded yourself with. Once you become conscious of these influences, you can begin to program yourself with positive emotions that have the power to heal and fill your life with abundance.

Stress and emotions not only affect organs like the heart, but they also create ripple effects that resonate down to the level of our mitochondrial DNA and even our chromosomes. Changes in our stress levels and emotional health can impact our cells' ability to create copies of mitochondrial DNA and can even shorten our *telomeres*, the ends of chromosomes that are affected by aging. Shortened telomeres are associated with aging, various cancers, and other health conditions.

As an example of this, people who suffer from depression have a higher risk of developing age-related conditions,[28] and they experience higher levels of inflammation in the body.[29]

From approximately ages fifteen to twenty-two, I was at a point in my life where I felt spiritually and mentally bankrupt, and I was searching for something to make me feel whole again. I had a tendency to internalize negative feelings. I didn't know how to talk about these emotions or express myself. I know the impact it can have on the physical body as well as the daily interaction with others; it is painful. I used

---

28 Jean-Philippe Gouin, Liisa V. Hantsoo, and Janice K. Kiecolt-Glaser, "Stress, Negative Emotions, and Inflammation," *The Oxford Handbook of Social Neuroscience*, September 2011.

29 Viktoriya Maydych, "The Interplay Between Stress, Inflammation, and Emotional Attention: Relevance for Depression," *Frontiers in Neuroscience*, April 24, 2019.

alcohol to numb myself from feeling these negative emotions, and the alcohol acted as a depressant as well.

I got myself out of depression through finding what foods caused inflammation, as well as by surfacing emotions and negative feelings I had jammed down deep inside of me. When I stopped drinking, I had no choice but to be confronted with the negative emotions and deal with them—and deal with them I did—and I never dealt with depression again.

The fear of dealing with darkness from the past is much greater than most people will ever think and the relief that can accompany it is life-changing. It is one of the reasons why confessions work, because when you release guilt, shame, anger, and fear from the brain and body, your energy can flow more freely.

At around twenty-two, I began a gratitude practice. Once I started this conscious daily spiritual practice, I began to see a profound psychic change.

Every day, I would start with a "daily dozen:" I'd write down a list of twelve things I was grateful for in that moment. I am not the first person to come up with this; people have been doing it for thousands of years. I later found through recent research that gratitude practices have shown to have a dramatic effect on people's lives, and it certainly had an impact on mine. Each day after writing my list, I noticed a shift in my energy, and even in my perception of my environment and my day. I would often wake up feeling irritable and angry, with my mind automatically ruminating on past experiences I was pissed off about. I would feel the weight of that heavy energy on my shoulders. I would get in the shower still feeling that irritation and negativity.

Over time, I consciously began to shift my thoughts and feelings. I rewired my brain and body to have a different experience when I get in the shower. It was a skill that took conscious attention. Now, I get into the shower and think, *Thank you, God—that I am lucky enough to live in a place where we have hot running water. There are millions of people who don't have this.* There is always something to be grateful for; we just have to look for it. Complaining is easy; finding the silver lining takes character. If we let our environments dictate our emotions, we become victims of our circumstances—but if we rise up and let our emotions and feelings dictate our environment, we have now made a conscious choice to take control of our environment, life, and health.

THE DAILY DOZEN GRATITUDE PRACTICE

The simple act of sitting down to focus on something you're grateful for can create huge changes in your energy. Think of that old saying, "It's hard to be hateful when you're grateful." You cannot have two emotions simultaneously. Each day, take a few minutes to write a list of twelve things you're extremely grateful for in the moment. If twelve is too many, just start off with a few things you can think of.

Then take a moment to pay attention to how your energy feels in your body, especially after a few weeks.

Feeling gratitude and joy in our bodies is a skill that we can practice. Just like brushing your teeth, you can do this simple practice each day to care for your mindset. A slight change in perception, from irritation to gratitude, can create a powerful new perspective in your life. To change your perspective is to change your reality. Sit back and watch how life will unfold in a more positive way.

A friend of mine tells a powerful story about gratitude and perspective. At one time in his life, my friend—let's call him Frank—had a real problem with alcohol, which he used to help escape his problems. He was on and off the wagon and always had excuses for why he picked up a drink again. One day, he was attending a support group for people who have a desire to stop drinking. He came into the meeting, sat down, and started complaining and giving excuses for why he'd begun to drink again. He had too many chores; work was demanding; his car broke down and he had to walk to work; he had problems with the wife...the list went on and on.

Before he could finish, an old timer in the group who I'll call Jim cut him off and said, "When I was newly sober, I lost a six-figure job and started pumping gas. Three years sober, I walked in on my wife having sex with my best friend. When I was seven years sober, my daughter was hit and killed by a drunk driver. When I was twenty years sober, I was diagnosed with a disease that will take years off my life. Not once did I drink over it. So the next time you come in here to give excuses as to why you drank, make sure my car isn't outside."

Frank was pissed off at what the old timer said, but the truth got his attention. The next day, Frank decided to pay Jim a visit. As Frank approached, he saw Jim scribbling something down, and when Jim was finished, he handed it over to Frank. "Read it," he said.

Frank looked at the list and Jim said: "Home. Wife. Job. Car. Health. You can walk. You can talk. You can dream. You can believe."

"All the things you complained about," Jim said, "that is your gratitude list. Your glasses are on backwards."

My buddy realized: Jim was right. Frank *had* a wife, and a car, and a house, and food on the table. He'd just been looking at the world from the negative point of view because his thinking was upside down.

Gratitude has the power to transform our mood and outlook because it fires up different parts of the brain than negative thoughts of guilt, shame, and anger.[30] The more we practice accessing these higher-vibration states, the more they change our experience, our perception, and our biology—which impacts our gene expression and influences our state of dis-ease or health.

CONNECTING THROUGH MEDITATION

In my experience, this one simple practice of holding an experience of joy, love, and gratitude in my mind and allowing the feeling to permeate every cell of my being and body creates a positive transformation for me and all of my clients. Start to practice holding this joy and gratitude in your own mind and see if it works for you. After all, what's the worst that can come of it? Even if it has no lasting effects for you, you'll have spent a few moments tapping into your own sense of joy and appreciation.

---

30 Arjun Walia, "Scientists Show How Gratitude Literally Alters the Human Heart and Molecular Structure of the Brain," *Collective Evolution*, February 14, 2019.

FILLING YOURSELF WITH LIQUID GOLDEN LIGHT

One of the best ways to identify the frequency you're operating at is to pay attention to your energy, thoughts, and feelings throughout the day. Take an inventory of the different emotions you experience and the energy that comes with them.

When do you feel heavy, lethargic, bogged down, or dispassionate?

When do you feel frustrated, irritated, or angry?

When do you feel fear, guilt, or shame? What triggered those feelings?

When do you feel peace, joy, love, and lightness?

In the times you need to feel lighter, you can shift your state with a simple guided meditation I use with my clients that is a mixture of many practices I learned along my healing journey. The goal is to get out of the conscious mind while doing this, and get into the limbic brain and alpha or theta states where reprogramming can begin. It is a skill that may take practice. The more you do it, the better you get, and the faster you shift your feelings and your life.

First, set an intention for what you would like to feel, understand, accept, let go of, or manifest. Then close your eyes and spend a few moments paying attention to your breath. Take 10 to 15 conscious breaths into the belly.

Picture a white light above your head. Allow that light to expand until it fills up your entire head. Imagine it filling up your brain stem down your spinal cord.

Then picture that golden liquid light pouring down your entire body. Imagine it running down your neck, your shoulders and your arms till the light shines out of your fingertips. Visualize it going down around your heart and pouring down your back behind your heart. Follow the light with your attention as you let it flow out through your torso, your hips, your legs, all the way down to your ankles and exits your toes.

I like to picture the cells themselves, inside the body, each lighting up like a lightbulb. Imagine each cell glowing, with a smiley face on every cell, and imagine them start to dance and jump around with joy like they are having a party.

You can put your hands over your heart and picture a time you felt deep gratitude for something in your life. Let that gratitude permeate every cell of your being; feel it as fully as you can. As you keep your attention on your body, you may feel it start to vibrate with the energy of your light and gratitude. You can even picture the feeling of love and gratitude pouring out of your heart and direct it to someone you love or want to send that energy to. They will receive it whether they are across the world or in the next room, and they will receive it whether they want to or not. A guy I know always says, "I love you and there's nothing you can do about it." He gets it—he is in charge of his emotions.

In one last step of the meditation, as you picture that golden light that fills up your whole being, you can shift your attention to the base of your spine. Hold in your mind that golden liquid light connecting to the center of the earth, connecting to a place that feels good, like a mother's love from Mother Earth.

Then picture the negative energy you're holding—any darkness, stress, or gunk in your body—getting absorbed into Mother Earth. Picture her pulling it away, removing all the darkness into the ground. As that negative energy flows out, imagine it being replaced by Mother Earth's love bouncing back up to you. Again, feel the love pouring into your soul, spirit, and cells.

This practice can help you release stuck emotions and cleans those thoughts and feelings from your mind, your body, and your spirit. You can stop carrying that baggage. Allow a feeling of lightness to come into your body in its place.

Mindfulness connects us to nature and the universal source of our energy that can charge the body with free energy, just like a rechargeable battery; that's what meditation is. It creates coherence with energy centers in the body as well as the heart and brain. That is a simple and quick practice you can do anywhere. You can play with the light as you please.

And the best part? We have access to this free energy at all times! It is there for you whenever you need it.

In Bruce Lipton's analogy of our energy being both an antenna and a broadcast, he describes how, even if the antenna breaks—even if we're not picking up certain frequencies—the broadcast is still there. By observing the frequencies we're picking up on, we can tune into the broadcast we want just like a radio station. Tune the channel as you please.

SYNCING WITH THE ENERGY OF OTHERS

In Lipton's analogy, we're both the antenna picking up frequencies, and we're also the broadcast. Each time we have a thought or feeling, we broadcast it through our thoughts, words, feelings, expressions, attitude, posture, dress, and actions. We feel this effect in the people we're around: when we spend time around people with whom we're on the same wavelength, we feel energized; we feel our energy elevated, we feel connected, and we feel good when our energy synchronizes with others.

The opposite can also be true. When the people who surround us are overweight, unhealthy, and chronically sick, not only will we pick up on that energy signature, but it becomes normal to us. As we start to pick up that energy, we may feel tired, sick, and cranky. We may start to complain more to fit in.

There's a joke in the mental health field, that before you get diagnosed with depression, make sure you're not surrounded by assholes. The people we surround ourselves with will either elevate us or bring us down, raise or lower our vibration.[31] Create a protective force field around you, a bubble

---

31 Nadia Vella, "Science Confirms that People Absorb Energy from Others," *Conscious Reminder*, 2016.

of positive energy, and you will begin to influence others or push away the negative people.

HACKING FREQUENCIES

Not only do our thoughts influence the frequencies of our cells, but we can also "hack" our cells with external frequencies. Researchers have been doing just that: a study on mice with Alzheimer's-like symptoms showed that their brain function could improve by exposing the mice to light and sound at specific frequencies. The neural connections in the brains of these mice had developed plaque, which was preventing those networks from firing efficiently.

Researchers found that frequencies that matched certain natural brain waves could break up plaque in the prefrontal cortex and hippocampus, crucial parts of the brain involved in cognition and memory.[32] Interestingly, the specific wavelength of sound the researchers used, 40 hertz, stimulates gamma waves in the brain. Gamma waves are among the highest-frequency waves in our brains, and they're associated with deep meditative states.

You can envision unhealthy cells as being clumped together in a mass of irregular cells. As we increase the energy and voltage of those cells, the activity of those cells increases. The cells that were out of harmony can be brought back into harmony, shake off the gunk or mucus that had them stuck, and increase the flow of energy and nutrients they need, making them healthier. In fact, a study showed that pulsed electromagnetic field (PEMF) therapy accelerates wound

---

32 Mike McRae, "Scientists 'Clear' Alzheimer's Plaque from Mice Using Only Light and Sound," *Science Alert*, March 15, 2019.

healing because the frequencies of PEMF stimulate cellular proliferation.[33] As the cells become healthier, so do we: we have increased energy, more mental clarity, better sleep, and faster recovery.

Inventor Jim Girard created a device he calls the BioCharger to stimulate cells. Research has been done to examine how cancer cells respond to electrical stimulation at different voltages.[34] Above a certain frequency, the study found, cancer cells begin to die off, and healthy cells proliferate. The BioCharger uses a combination of PEMF therapy, photon therapy, sound vibration, and standard magnetic therapy to "speak" to the body's cells, charge them, and bring them in tune with the natural frequency they need. For example, all your kidney cells vibrate together at a certain frequency, and PEMF can bring the kidneys back in harmony if they were off.

Through these four technologies, Girard could make subtle adjustments to the frequencies of waves being directed at the body. Each of the organ and brain centers has its own frequency, and he could create "recipes" that target specific areas in the body.

To understand how cells respond to frequencies, Girard says to think of a pair of tuning forks. If they're tuned to the same frequency, and I strike one, he says, "I could, through sympathetic vibration, cause the other tuning fork to ring." In an interview with me, Girard said the same thing happens to

33 Ozan Karaman, et al, "Comparative Assessment of Pulsed Electromagnetic Fields (PEMF) and Pulsed Radio Frequency Energy (PRFE) on an *In Vitro* Wound Healing Model," *International Journal of Applied Electromagnetics and Mechanics*, July 9, 2018, 57(4): 427-437.

34 Jeffrey Roberts, "Researchers Demonstrate How Cancer Cells Are Obliterated by Resonant Frequencies," *Collective Evolution*, January 21, 2016.

cells. With the BioCharger, "I generate that particular harmonic on a cellular level of frequency. I can begin to 'ring' that cell and transfer energy, much like you could transfer the energy of a voice through a radio signal."[35] The frequency charges up the cell, giving it the energy it needs to repair.

I began experimenting with these technologies and discovered these therapies worked for me. Science aside, nothing speaks louder than results. After my first session, my body expelled mucus, one of the main causes of disease. I also experienced a huge increase in energy—more than I'd had in years. I not only saw huge improvements in my own health, but I heard from others who experienced deep healing after a single session with the BioCharger or PEMF therapy. For example, I heard from people who were able to stop taking sleeping pills they'd been on for two years, and they slept better than ever.

There are recipes that help with Lyme disease, parasites, exercise recovery, individual organs, autoimmunity, PTSD, autism, meditation—the list goes on and on, because every organ, every part of the brain, and every organism vibrates at a specific frequency.

As Nikola Tesla famously said: "If you want to know the secrets of the universe, study frequency, vibration, and energy." These subtle energies, in the form of frequency that surrounds us in nature, have the power to bring us back into harmony. We use a Biocharger at EarthFIT and combine it with breathwork and exercise to maximize results, healing, and recovery. That is another simple healing hack: doing

---

35   Jim Girard, in conversation with the author, June 4, 2019.

breathwork (like the exercises we'll describe in the next chapter) with PEMF can enhance results.

SOUND MEDITATION

As we look at the role of frequency in our wellbeing, it's no surprise that sound can play a powerful role in assisting the healing process or reharmonizing the body.

The BioCharger uses specific wavelengths of sound to target particular systems of the body. A similar device, the AmpCoil, uses sound therapy as well as PEMF to stimulate the healing process. You can speak directly into a biofeedback tool, and by analyzing your voice, the AmpCoil can tell which areas of the body are the highest priority for healing, as it pertains to organ systems, nutrition, toxins, poison, parasites, microbes.

This technology was designed specifically for people with Lyme disease and autoimmune conditions but helps with a whole range of other health issues. I have been using the AmpCoil for over two years now. One of the first things I used it for was a sleep journey. I didn't realize how terrible my sleep was because of my health issues, but when I set the AmpCoil to a deep sleep program, I could feel it activating specific parts of my brain that may have been malfunctioning, and I drifted into a deep sleep like I hadn't in years.

The idea behind these devices is that specific harmonies have healing effects for different parts of the body or even brain centers. We feel the effects of different harmonies just from specific vibration. You don't need complex devices like the BioCharger or an AmpCoil to create these effects; you can access these wavelengths through simpler methods, in the form of sound meditation, which uses crystal bowls and other instruments to help reach a deep state of meditation.

I visited a sound meditation center in Scottsdale, Arizona, where the practitioners use crystal bowls and other objects to create specific tones and harmonies, and I had one of the best restorative meditations. I also visited a high-level sound healer and did a one-on-one session. The session was about three hundred dollars, and it was well worth it. This sound healer put a vibration of 432 megahertz on my back. I sat in a hammock staring at a mesmerizing image on the wall that seemed to be pulsing with movement. In the meditation room were the same bowls ringing around me, and the vibration of these tools put me in the deepest meditative state; I felt like I had gone to another universe and back. It took me awhile to catch my bearings. Sound has the power to bring us—quite literally—back into harmony.

There is also a new field that has emerged called sonogenetics, in which sound waves are used to control neural activity in the brain only by using sound frequency. Recent research indicates that simply drumming accelerates healing. In a study conducted by Barry Bitman, neurologist and president of the Yamaha Music and Wellness Institute, blood samples were drawn from participants after they'd participated in an hour-long drumming session. The blood tests showed a decrease in stress hormones and an increase in natural T-cells that help the body combat viruses and cancers.[36] Sound and vibration can be harnessed as healing therapies.

Throughout this book, we'll continue to look at how our

---

36 Christiane Northrup, "10 Health Reasons to Start Drumming," *DrNorthrup.com*, March 21, 2016.

thoughts, feelings, and frequencies influence all the systems of our bodies, and I'll offer the healing hacks I've learned after studying numerous healers from all over the world for over a decade. In the following chapters, I touch on a few specific healers that you benefit from knowing about if you don't already. When I tell people about what some of these healers have been able to heal, many people don't even believe how effective their methods can be. I offer these techniques for you to try, and in the end, your best evidence for what works for you is your own experience and ultimately how you feel.

THE HACKS

At the end of each chapter, I'll offer a quick list of the practices mentioned so you can keep a library of techniques to return to and practice along your own healing journey. We'll break these down into the "Accessible Methods," which include low-cost and beginner practices, "Advanced Methods," which are higher cost or for more experienced practitioners, and "Things to Consider Avoiding," which sums up any cautions or common habits to break. You can use these practices to jumpstart your healing in all the different areas of your life.

Accessible Methods
- Inventory your stories
- Daily dozen gratitude list
- Golden light meditation
- Drumming circles

Advanced Methods
- The BioCharger and AmpCoil

- Other Pulsed electromagnetic field (PEMF) therapies
- Sound meditation

Things to Consider Avoiding

- Consider not judging yourself if you have negative feelings. The fact that you are aware they are there is a *huge* win and a powerful step in the right direction. We are human and will have emotions that range from low to high, but when we can pinpoint the negative emotions, process them, and shift them, then we are now in control of what we manifest.

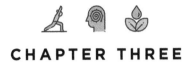

CHAPTER THREE

THE IMPORTANCE OF OXYGEN

While figuring out how to heal my ailments, through experimentation I noticed doing deep breathing techniques made a dramatic impact on how I felt. I had seen how breathing helped people with anxiety and a variety of other conditions, so I explored numerous techniques and created my own just through playing around with what made me feel better. When I practiced deep inhalations and breath holds, I noticed my anxiety would instantly go down, and I felt more relaxed and it seemed that whatever was taking over my body was held at bay for the time being. I was dealing with the persistent, stabbing sensation in the back of my head that I described earlier, but I found the sensation would be relieved when I took deep breaths.

I came across the work of Wim Hof, a pioneer of mindset, cold exposure, and breathing techniques. After following along to online videos of his method, I thought, *Wow! These results are next level* (and I eventually came to find out that I wasn't even doing the method correctly). Since I was already in health and fitness and all about getting results in the safest, fastest, and most effective way, naturally I knew this was something I had to dive deeper into.

I began studying with Wim Hof because it was clear his technique was far superior to anything I'd previously experienced when it came to breathwork. It had a powerful physiological effect, greater than anything I had ever felt previously, and I could literally feel the healing happening in my body in *real time*. I made the decision (and the investment) to work with him in person. It was one of the best decisions I have ever made. At that point, I had already worked with and studied from some of the best doctors and trainers in the world—and after watching Wim on TV I could recognize he was the real deal.

Wim Hof was nicknamed "the Iceman" when he became famous for numerous feats such as being able to withstand ice baths for almost two hours, without inducing hypothermia. During these ice bath sessions, sometimes his body temp would drop to 88 degrees—but through his breathing and meditation techniques, he was able to heat his own body back up naturally, which was previously thought to be impossible. He climbed Mount Kilimanjaro three times in record pace, wearing only shorts. His last ascent took thirty-one hours, while the typical ascent takes five to seven days. Even crazier, he was able to coach a group of people who had chronic illnesses through the climb; his participants had diseases like Lyme and Crohn's, and they had no mountaineering experience.

He developed his technique by going out in extreme environments in nature, doing breathwork, cold immersion, and meditation, and seeing how his body responded. He followed his intuition. When he was eighteen, he decided to chop a hole in the ice and submerge his whole body. Both in the documentary on Hof and in workshops I attended, Wim recollected that this is where he met God and began his journey.

Since then, he has run a half marathon barefoot in ice and snow above the Arctic Circle; he swam fifty meters under layers of ice with water temps below freezing; he ran a marathon in sandals in the desert in Africa without drinking water. While exploring his own body's responses to these extremes, he was able to develop control and have influence on his body's thermoregulation, and autonomic nervous and immune systems, which was previously thought to be impossible.

Hof was demonstrating control over body systems that were considered automatic and unconscious, and the scientific community set up numerous studies to investigate his abilities.

A 2012 study revealed the true power of this method. At Radbaud University, they tested Wim's inflammatory response and looked at levels of cytokines in his blood. (Cytokines are substances released by cells of the immune system that are inflammatory markers. By measuring cytokines in the blood, we can measure the actions of the immune system.) They injected him with lipopolysaccharides (LPS), an inert endotoxin found in harmful bacteria like *E. coli*. When injected into test subjects, the LPS doesn't replicate to cause disease, but it does give people temporary flu-like symptoms as their bodies recognize the foreign invaders and provoke an inflammatory response. Typically, test subjects would get chills and shakes, and researchers would see their cytokine levels go up. Because of these ill effects, scientists joke that LPS stands for "little pieces of shit"—because, in essence, that is what they are.

After researchers injected LPS into Hof, he performed his

breathing and meditation techniques. The result? He had none of the same symptoms. At most, he reported being a little headachy.

While the researchers were amazed by this result, they considered Hof to be an anomaly. He protested that he wasn't—and that he could replicate this effect by training others how to control their immune response.

In 2014, the researchers set up a second experiment: they divided a group of twenty-four volunteers into a group of twelve individuals who would be trained in Wim Hof's method, and a group of twelve who would remain untrained controls. Both groups were injected with LPS. The twelve volunteers who had been trained in the breathing and meditation technique by Hof demonstrated the same response that Hof did. This was one of the first-ever studies to demonstrate that we can have an influence on our innate immune system.[37]

I came across Wim Hof's techniques at a much-needed point in my healing journey. At that time, I was experiencing symptoms in my nerves: I had numbness in my left arm, and shooting pains and numbness down my left leg.

After feeling fatigued and sick for so long, depression had set in, so much so that I couldn't function. I'd tried everything I could think of, and some of the methods had made matters worse: the numbness had started after doing a sauna niacin

---

37 Henriet van Middendorp, Matthijs Kox, Peter Pickkers, and Andrea W. M. Evers, "The Role of Outcome Expectancies for a Training Program Consisting of Meditation, Breathing Exercises, and Cold Exposure on the Response to Endotoxin Administration: a Proof-of-Principle Study," *Clinical Rheumatology*, July 21, 2015, 35: 1081-85.

detox, and I'd had a full-blown panic attack after experimenting with medical marijuana oil in hopes that it would provide some healing and relief, but it only made matters worse. I no longer had the energy and drive to push through the pain I'd had for so long. I had again reached a point where I had no desire to live. I had even become convinced that I was going to die very early. I fantasized about selling my business (a process I actually started), going to live in Costa Rica, and just letting go. No one knew what I was going through; I hadn't told anyone how bad my mental state was. Finally, one day, I broke down and told a mentor what I was going through. He wondered if I was exaggerating, but it really was that bad. It was a relief to tell someone and let go of those negative feelings I'd stored up. I just wanted relief from the constant pain and fatigue.

When I came across YouTube videos describing Wim Hof's method, I started practicing his sequence for breathwork. I would take deep, full breaths and hold them, and visualize squeezing the oxygen of that breath into my head. After practicing this technique, I felt better: I had less inflammation, more energy, better physical flexibility, and mobility, and I noticed my brain was functioning better. I was happier. Most importantly, I felt relief.

Just like the difference between exercising to a video and working with a personal trainer, I knew I would get so much more out of working with Hof face-to-face in real time. I signed up for my first retreat to practice with him in Spain.

My sessions on that retreat were profound experiences. We did breathing techniques designed to decalcify the pineal gland in the brain—which is sometimes referred to as the "third eye" or the "seat of the soul"—and I could feel my brain centers opening up. We were practicing outside, and I felt connected to the earth and connected to the people with me. We were all searching for similar things. I knew this was my tribe. I was reconnecting to nature, to my true self, and to other like-minded people.

The retreat was so impactful I went on to become an instructor in the Wim Hof method. As a fitness professional for fifteen years with some of the best education the world has to offer, I get presented with endless certification and I am very picky about where I invest my time and energy, but this was a no-brainer for me. This practice, I knew, could help others heal like it had for me and I have seen unreal changes happen for my clients in just one session. But it can also help others with performance, sleep, inflammation, injury, and exercise recovery. The list goes on and on.

LEARNING HOW TO BREATHE

Just as infants do, we take belly breaths when we're relaxed. These deep breaths stimulate the parasympathetic nervous system, where we begin to rest and digest. Our cortisol levels drop, our pupils constrict, and we secrete more saliva and stomach acid to prepare for digestion. The bronchioles in our lungs constrict because we don't have as much demand on them as when we're in fight or flight.

But as you might expect, modern life has us living in sympathetic nervous system mode much of the time. When we're stressed, our breathing is shallow. Our bronchioles dilate, and blood flows to the extremities to prepare us to take action in fight or flight.

Whether we're actually engaging in a fight or fleeing a physical threat is irrelevant; the responses still play out in our physiology because the brainstem tells the rest of the body that a threat is imminent. These responses even affect our posture: for example, someone who has a persistent fight response can develop the rounded-in shoulders and protective posture of a boxer. A person who is constantly in flight typically has strong and bigger legs because blood is constantly sent in that direction ready to flee.

When we take constricted, shallow breaths all day every day, we reduce the amount of oxygen to every cell in the body. The number-one threat to the body is lack of oxygen (and it also could be said, an improper ratio of carbon dioxide to oxygen)—if we don't have oxygen for even a few minutes, we die. Without oxygen, the mitochondria of our cells are unable to fire, and thus the cells lose energy. The effects cascade from there: when people live in extreme stress for long periods of time, they experience adrenal fatigue, illness, and disease.

Breathing techniques are one of the fastest, lowest-hanging fruit to help us change our health dramatically. Deep breathing helps us tone the *vagus nerve*, also known as the "wandering" nerve or the tenth cranial nerve, which is responsible for activating our parasympathetic nervous system.[38] The vagus nerve runs from our brain down around the heart and out through the arms, down to the stomach, and into the digestive system. Along this path it branches out to all the parts of our body like the roots of a tree—a reflection of the nature that we are part of. Good vagal tone leads to good health: the more vagal tone we have, the better the body is

---

38 Christopher Bergland, "Vagus Nerve Stimulation Dramatically Reduces Inflammation,"
    Psychology Today, July 6, 2016.

able to cope with stress, as well as stimulate healing. When you stimulate the vagus nerve, you send information to your body that it is time to de-stress, relax, and go into recovery mode. It is also through the parasympathetic nervous system that love, peace, and happiness can be activated.

QUICK TIPS TO IMPROVE VAGAL TONE

1. Practice controlled, deep, slow, belly breathing.
2. Cold exposure like cold showers, cold plunges, or any acute cold exposure has been proven to activate the vagus nerve, and we'll discuss cold exposure in more depth later in this chapter. Splashing cold water on the face is a simple and easy way to activate the vagus nerve.
3. Chanting, singing, and humming all stimulate the vagus nerve.
4. Research on meditation shows that meditation improves vagal tone, reducing "fight or flight" activity in the nervous system, while increasing positive emotions.[39]
5. Exercise.
6. Boost your connections with others through socialization and laughter.
7. Get a massage.
8. Because the vagus nerve connects the gut to the brain, good gut bacteria (through a live food diet and probiotics) improves vagal tone and mood.

---

39 Jordan Fallis, "How to Stimulate Your Vagus Nerve for Better Mental Health," *Optimal Living Dynamics*, August 24, 2019.

9. Omega 3 Fatty acids, fatty acids, and cholesterol are nerve and brain insulators and cannot be produced by the body. Supplementation of these nutrients helps with cognitive decline and the repairing of the blood brain barrier.

USING BREATH TO CONNECT

After I'd become a Wim Hof instructor, I began to use breathwork at EarthFIT. One of our clients, Barbara, had been training at EarthFIT for eight or so years. Just before she'd come to train at EarthFIT for the first time, she'd lost her husband. In the years since, Barbara had not been able to fully release her grief.

Barbara came to a Wim Hof Method workshop that I held at EarthFIT, and as she started on the breathing exercises she was overcome by intense emotion. She started crying, and she said later that she felt she was able to release a lot of the negative emotions she'd had around her husband's death. For the first time in eight or nine years, she said she had more emotional healing in one session than she'd had in the past eight to nine years and was puzzled by the profound impact.

BREATHWORK RELEASES EMOTIONS

Negative feelings like grief, anger, and shame get trapped in our bodies. They get stuck in our nervous system and trapped in our brains like honey on a honeycomb. We carry these emotions around with us all the time.

Just by using oxygen, we can reconnect with those places in our bodies and minds that we've shut down and become disconnected from. Our breath allows us to open up the flow of energy through our systems, so that we can release negative or unwanted feelings, and this stimulates the healing process. Physical symptoms can and will manifest from unchecked and unexpressed emotions.

We can see physical signs when this energy begins to be released. At our training facility, I was working with another client on breathwork when her legs began to shake. I could tell this was a big response from her nervous system. "I don't know what just happened," she said, "I feel like I'm going to cry." I explained to her that this was a normal part of the process, and that she was releasing negative emotions and feelings deep in the nervous system. I encouraged her to cry. She went in the bathroom, and when she came back out after she was done crying, she said, "That was life changing."

BREATHWORK RELIEVES STRESS

Breathwork helps us with big, emotional release, but it can also help us with small, daily stressors. Another client I worked with at our Wim Hof Retreat in Costa Rica was a coffee addict. Coffee was one of the ways he dealt with feeling stressed out all the time, and it also kept him in sympathetic mode. He wasn't breathing properly—when we began working together, he literally had to be taught how to belly breathe again, and breathe deeply into his diaphragm. We did strength exercises to get his belly and diaphragm activated. The first thing he asked in the morning before the breathing exercise was, "Is there coffee?"

"No," I said, "there's no coffee for you. It's not recommended when you're practicing this kind of breath work."

"Oh my god," he said, and his face fell. He believed he needed coffee to function, and he was stressed out about the thought of pushing through the day without it.

By the end of the retreat, he was dumbfounded that he'd had no coffee the entire time—and he felt amazing. He had no headaches, no irritability, and contrary to what he'd been afraid of, he felt energized and happy every day—and this was all a result of the Wim Hof breathing technique. Withdrawals from caffeine are caused by expanding blood vessels in the brain. When we consume coffee, caffeine causes the blood vessels to narrow, and when we stop drinking it, the blood vessels expand, creating an experience known as a "coffee headache." The Wim Hof breathing can help this by regulating the inflammatory markers and increasing the natural endocannabinoids and opioids in the system to reduce pain and regulate blood pressure.

BREATHWORK INCREASES MOBILITY

Like we saw earlier, a lack of oxygen in addition to low carbon dioxide causes stress to the body and creates an unconscious signal of threat. The more you feel threatened, the more rigid and restricted your movement will be. Mobility and flexibility will be drastically reduced, and you can develop shoulder pain, back pain, or other bodily pain from this immobility and lack of oxygen. Chronic reduction in oxygen and hydration can also drastically affect connective tissue, which encases all the muscles of the body.

You can see the effects oxygen has on your mobility with a simple test. Sit down, straighten your legs out in front of you, and reach for your toes. Note how far you get. Then, take in about ten deep belly breaths (or practice the Wim Hof method that appears later in this chapter), and do the sit and reach test again. You may be amazed at how much more limber you are after breathing deeply.

HOW OXYGEN HEALS

Science is still trying to catch up in terms of understanding what makes breathwork such a powerful healing tool, but some studies are beginning to show that the lungs are doing far more for the health of many of our body's systems than was previously thought.

A 2017 study on mice at the University of California San Francisco revealed that lungs aren't solely used for respiration. Through video microscopy of living mice lungs, researchers found that the lungs also play a role in producing blood. While it was previously understood that platelets and other blood components were produced in bone marrow, the study found that the lungs produced more than half of the mice's blood platelets, and they also contained stem cells that could produce other components.[40]

The oxygen we take in with each breath becomes the pump and driver for every function of the cell, and every function of the body. When we take deep breaths, we hyperoxygenate the body. Oxygen levels rise and carbon dioxide levels drop. This increases alkalinity in the body, so much so that you can measure the effect on an alkaline test strip. In our retreats in Costa Rica, we have people pee on a test strip before the

---

40 Lefrançais, Emma, et al, "The Lung is a Site of Platelet Biogenesis and a Reservoir for Haematopoietic Progenitors," *Nature*, 2017, 544: 105-109.

breathing sessions and after to see the change in pH levels. Sometimes, seeing is believing.

This is important because the rise in oxygen—and therefore alkalinity—helps expel acids and mucus in the body, which is where pathogens, bacteria, and viruses like to thrive. People promote alkaline diets and alkaline water for their health benefits, and we'll discuss both in more depth in chapter five, but the fastest and easiest way to increase alkalinity in the body is simply through breathing.

If you do deep breathing before anaerobic training, you'll perform better because you've hyperoxygenated the body. After anaerobic training, when lactic acid levels are high, the Wim Hof method can help flush lactic acid faster from the body as well. Breathwork before and after exercise leads to better performance and better recovery time.

HOW AEROBIC AND ANAEROBIC CONDITIONING WORKS

Aerobic training refers to exercises and activities that utilize oxygen for energy. By American College of Sports Medicine guidelines, aerobic training utilizes large muscle groups that can be maintained continuously and is rhythmic in nature such as dancing, cycling, hiking, jogging/long distance running, swimming, and walking—activities of low to medium intensity that typically last twenty minutes or longer. This kind of exercise creates cardiovascular conditioning, which can be measured by assessing aerobic capacity, or the cardiorespiratory system's ability to supply oxygen in tandem with the skeletal muscles' ability to utilize oxygen.

Anaerobic training is short in duration and a much higher intensity than aerobic training, typically uses different muscle fiber types, too, and the body taps into a different energy system utilizing energy within the contracting muscles rather than the inhaled oxygen as an energy source. In the most basic sense, anaerobic training causes the body's cells to switch from using oxygen for fuel to using glycogen. Essentially, this type of exercise is fueled by sugars or energy that is readily available in your muscles. Typically, an anaerobic activity lasts for one to three minutes and utilizes fast-twitch muscle fibers used in such exercises as sprinting, jumping, or high-intensity interval training (HIIT). As your body burns through the fuel in the muscles, lactic acid can build up in the body. If you were to push yourself until you couldn't go any longer, your body would stop when it reaches a lactic acid threshold. You know this lactic acid threshold when you feel it: your body feels completely burned out and you can't run anymore. Think of a sprinter who runs two laps full out, and then falls to the ground afterward—many times they've hit their lactic acid threshold.

Because anaerobic activity happens without oxygen, you can create an oxygen deficit in the body easier with anaerobic training. When you have created an oxygen deficit, your body needs to take in more oxygen to replenish and restore the body back to homeostasis, which includes but is not limited to: reoxygenating the blood, decreasing body temperature, and returning to normal blood pressure and heart and breathing rates. During this phase, the amount of oxygen the body consumes after exercise over the pre-exercise baseline oxygen consumption level is called *excess post-exercise oxygen consumption* (EPOC). Basically, during intense exercises we use more oxygen post workout than during the actual workout. As you take in more oxygen during the EPOC phase such as when performing breathwork, that extra oxygen speeds up the healing and recovery process by bringing the oxygen levels back faster and removing the acids from the muscles faster. Hyperbaric oxygen chambers help with post exercise recovery for the same reasons, but with breathwork, you can do it anywhere any time. Research has indicated that oxygen consumption can be increased up to twenty-four hours post exercise, which also translates to increased caloric burn for those interested in fat burning.

IMPROVING YOUR HEART RATE VARIABILITY THROUGH BREATHING

Heart rate variability (HRV) has gained a lot of attention for its association with recovery, readiness, and life longevity. HRV is a measure of the variation of your heartrate within a given time frame. It is just one indicator of your overall health, recovery, and readiness. Cardiovascular training can help to improve your HRV.

Breathwork alone is cardio training, and I have seen it have massive impact on HRV by using the emWave, a heart rate rhythm monitor by HeartMath, to monitor my heart rate before and after a breathing session. (The Oura Ring activity tracker is another tool that can measure HRV.) When I was at my advanced Wim Hof certification in LA, I was talking with Wim when a doctor who was attending came up to Wim and started telling him that she tested HRV while using the breathing method, and when she saw it instantly improve after a session, she knew that there had to be something powerful to the technique. She said it was one of the main catalysts for her getting the Wim Hof Method certification.

BREATHING TECHNIQUES

When practicing breathwork, it's important to activate your diaphragm, which is one of the most important muscles in the body, since it not only pulls air into the lungs, but also massages all the internal organs.

A good position to fully activate the diaphragm is to lay down on your back with your knees bent so that your pelvis, diaphragm and neck are in alignment. When they are all in alignment, you will fully activate the diaphragm. Take deep breaths and pay attention to how your diaphragm expands and contracts.

Below are a few breathing techniques that are simple to practice when you're beginning a breathwork practice.

BUTEYKO BREATHING

Russian scientist Konstantin Buteyko was assigned to monitor the breathing patterns of diseased patients when to his surprise, he noticed that patients tended to deepen their breathing as death approached. This observation provided a foundation for the idea that "over-breathing" depletes carbon dioxide levels, which in turn causes oxygen starvation in tissues and spasms in the blood vessels, resulting in health issues.

Buteyko suggested breathing very lightly and calmly through the nose to balance out levels of oxygen and carbon dioxide and increase oxygenation of organs, tissues, and the brain. Later in this chapter, we'll look at the Wim Hof Method, which gets the same results in a completely different way. Buteyko breathing can be incorporated as a lifestyle change, while the Wim Hof Method is similar to a workout for the breath. Buteyko breathing is for people who want to walk; the Wim Hof Method is for those who want to sprint.

BOX BREATHING

This breathwork technique is great for stress control and is used by Navy SEALS before sleep, during training sessions, and during stressful events.

To practice this method, exhale slowly over a count of four seconds, hold your breath for four seconds, inhale slowly over four seconds, and hold your breath for four seconds. Repeat for as long as you feel comfortable. You can extend the number of counts for this exercise depending on how your body feels.

THE WIM HOF METHOD

While we refer to this set of breathing techniques as "the Wim Hof method," (WHM) it's worth noting that Wim had no method—he just went out and played in nature. This breathing technique arose from what he observed about his own body. Similarly, as you practice breathwork, it's important to observe how your own body responds. You can adapt this method and do a lot of different, amazing things. Breathwork can also get very advanced and potentially dangerous because of how deeply it can influence our systems, so it's important to stay connected to your own experience as you practice. When I truly learned this method's potential, it was the first time that I felt I had real control over my body, meaning it was the first time that I felt I was able to fight off whatever it was that was causing me so many physical and mental health issues.

To practice the basic method, first find a comfortable and safe environment where you can sit or lie down as you practice. Breathwork can make you dizzy or lightheaded, so it's important never to practice while you're driving, standing, swimming, operating heavy machinery, or in any other environment that could put you at risk, such as standing near a pool. I have heard of a very experienced practitioner doing a specific breathing technique while standing on a bridge, and the practitioner passed out and fell into the river. It's important to take precautions for your safety.

The basic process is simple: You begin by taking thirty to fifty deep breaths. Fully inhale on each breath, taking the air in like a wave from your belly, into your chest, into your head. Exhale about halfway out and breathe in deeply again. And as Wim says, "you can use any hole" to breathe in—the mouth or nose—but for beginners, the nose is typically recommended. At the end of this breathing cycle, exhale fully and hold your breath out for as long as your body feels comfortable—this could be several seconds to a couple of minutes.

Never force anything. When your body signals for you to inhale, take a deep breath in. Hold the inhalation for ten to fifteen seconds, as long as your body feels comfortable. When your body signals for you to breathe out, exhale and return to normal breathing. After you've completed a cycle of breath, you can repeat for several rounds of this breathing. The retention helps your body become more efficient at utilizing oxygen as well as numerous other benefits which we go deeper into.

Let's break down that process, and the effect it has on the body, one step at a time.

Some people refer to the first thirty to fifty fast belly breaths as "controlled hyperventilation," but hyperventilation often has negative connotations with shallow, panicked breathing that is not within our control. Instead, these breaths should be deep—think of this as "superventilation," as you are in control. As you take each breath in, make sure you're activating your diaphragm, which is one of the most important muscles in the body. Each time you take a deep breath in, imagine the diaphragm opening up like a balloon under the ribcage, and then fill up your lungs fully. The pressure from the diaphragm actually massages your internal organs. Deep, full-belly breaths hyperoxygenate the body.

On each exhalation, focus on breathing out about fifty percent of your breath. This is a good starting point to get used to the pace and technique of the breath. Once you're used to this rapid deep breathing, you can play with how deep the exhalations are. Try exhaling seventy-five percent of your breath on each one, and see the different effect it has. The deeper you exhale, the more you'll slow your breath down. On the other hand, there are times I've done this technique with instructors where we made our breath shallower, only exhaling about twenty-five percent of the way, and that makes those breaths super rapid. Each of these breathing styles has different effects that we can feel in the nervous system.

The key, as you experiment with how these breaths feel, is to stay as relaxed as possible on the exhale. The more relaxed you can be, the more oxygen will get to the cells. Often, when people first learn this technique, they tend to stay tense and tight because they think they have to breathe so fast and intense—but that tension constricts the cells and prevents energy and oxygen from going into the cells. Maintain a relaxed rhythm and flow of energy, so that you can enjoy the process rather than push it to a degree that feels super intense. The more you practice, you'll find the easier it is to relax, and you'll feel that your energy is more free-flowing.

Pay attention to how you feel the breath go into your head. Some people feel a slight tingling or buzzing. Others feel other sensations in their skull or sinuses, or they may notice a light ringing in their ears. Your hands may curl into "T-Rex hands" from the vasoconstriction of the super oxygenation. You may experience sensations in other parts of your body as well, such as a spot where you've had an injury or trauma. These sensations may be an indicator that healing is taking place in that area. Once you begin to feel dizzy or lightheaded, take one last full breath in, then exhale fully, and hold the exhalation out.

As you hold your breath out, your body will automatically try to get back to homeostasis. As you took those deep, fast breaths, your oxygen levels went up and carbon dioxide levels went down; now, as you hold your breath with no oxygen in the lungs, the body begins to balance out the systems as carbon dioxide levels rise. The lungs and the body will naturally sound off alarm signals. This begins a cascade of physiological events: epinephrine and norepinephrine are released and your body goes into flight or fight. The body releases adrenaline—more than if you were going to go bungee jumping the first time. This breathwork can also trigger the endocannabinoid system and the opioid system, releasing neurochemicals and hormones that reduce pain and help with the healing process.

Carbon dioxide levels rise as you hold your breath out, and

this creates crucial benefits for the body. Carbon dioxide plays an important role in brachial dilation (expansion of the airways), vasodilation (expansion of the arteries), muscle relaxation, pH regulation, tissue healing, red blood cell production, and the ability of red blood cells to carry more oxygen. It relaxes the alveoli in the lungs to soothe hyperventilation, and it also stabilizes the nerves and has a calming, sedative effect on the cells. Our most effective antioxidants are oxygen and carbon dioxide, and breathwork and exercise are the most effective methods of flushing free radicals from the body.

The length of time to hold the exhalation (with the lungs completely empty) will depend on the person and will change and vary per person and situation. It's okay to hold your breath out for just twenty to thirty seconds at the beginning of your practice while you are adapting. Around one minute is where the magic happens, and where most of the benefit of this breathing technique lies. Some people can hold their breath with no oxygen in the lungs for up to three, four, or even five minutes. Since you can release adrenaline at will during breathwork, this simple exercise reveals that you have voluntary influence over your autonomic nervous system.

When you feel you need to take a deep breath in, take your next inhale and hold it for ten to fifteen seconds. It's important to never force your breath, and to follow your body's signals for how many breaths to take, how long to hold your exhale, and when to return to breathing normally.

It's important to note that you can over-oxygenate your body with this exercise, which can make you feel dizzy and faint.

It's crucial to keep your awareness on your body and not force anything.

Doing breathwork by yourself will reap benefits; working with a professional can be life changing. A professional can help you refine your technique and monitor the effects.

BREATHING AND CONTRACTION

When you've practiced this breath for a while and become familiar and comfortable with it, you can begin to expand on the technique. One additional step I do is to take a full deep breath in and "squeeze" oxygen to areas of my body that need it. Complete the thirty to fifty deep breaths as described earlier, and then exhale fully. Hold the exhale and squeeze or tense up any muscles that may need a little bit of love and attention: your glutes, your back, your neck muscles, and your shoulders are easy muscle groups to target. As you hold the exhale and squeeze these muscles, your arteries will contract and so will your cells. For example, if your intestines need some love, suck in the belly around the area where you want to send more oxygen. The more you deprive and use up the oxygen faster, the more oxygen the body will demand when you take that deep breath in after the retention.

When you feel you need to take a breath in, inhale fully. Your arteries will now expand, and as you hold your inhale, you can "push" blood, energy and oxygen to the muscle groups and areas you're targeting: Imagine like a tube of toothpaste, you are squeezing the oxygen to any body part that needs particular attention, but this time the cells are screaming for oxygen because they have been deprived more than usual. They will happily intake more oxygen to make up for it.

OXYGEN LEVELS

The amount of oxygen the body needs varies depending on the activity or situation. Exercise and altitude changes, for example, change the body's oxygen demands. If the body is carrying normal amounts of oxygen, the blood cells are referred to as "saturated." Too much and too little oxygen in the blood can have unwanted consequences, but the body can adapt. The more versatile or adaptable the body is to change, the stronger the organism is.

We can monitor oxygen levels with a little tool such as a pulse oximeter. This sensor clips to the fingers and measures heart rate and oxygen levels. Normal oxygen saturation levels are typically ninety-five to one hundred percent. Oxygen saturation levels below eighty percent can compromise organs; low levels usually need to be addressed instantly. When doing the Wim Hof retention, we have seen blood oxygen levels go below sixty percent, which is considered clinically dead. But this is possible—and causes no issues—because of what is believed to be oversaturation of blood oxygen levels from the breathwork and the alkalinity of the blood. With the Wim Hof training, you are training the body to deal with extreme situations and become more efficient with oxygen, to the point where evidence suggests that people who engage in acute hypoxia training may be able to increase the survival rate of heart attacks dramatically: a promising non-pharmacological way for prevention and treatment of cardiovascular disease.[41]

---

41 "Hypoxia Training Suppresses Harmful Cardiac Nitric Oxide Production During Heart Attack,"
    Society for Experimental Biology and Medicine, May 27, 2008.

ALTITUDE TRAINING

For some people, simply going up a mountain may be enough for the body to adapt and increase oxygen efficiency. Others can exercise at altitude to increase their performance, an effect that has been used by athletes for a long time. In fact, a method of "blood doping" involves training at high altitudes, drawing and storing blood, and injecting the highly oxygenated blood before a race. The increased oxygen creates such a performance boost that blood doping has been banned in competitions.

INTERMITTENT HYPOXIA THERAPY

It's possible to mimic the same effects of altitude training with devices that hook up to the mouth and restrict oxygen to simulate breathing at high altitude. In response to the low-oxygen environment, the body increases the activity of neurotransmitters like serotonin and stimulates the brain and spinal cord. Because of these effects, intermittent hypoxia therapy is being investigated for its ability to help spinal cord injuries and respiratory issues.[42] In Russia, doctors have used intermittent hypoxia training for decades to improve memory, brain function, circulation, red blood cell and stem cell production, and production of cancer-protecting proteins. Intermittent hypoxia training can benefit inflammatory conditions such as Alzheimer's, Parkinson's, dementia, neurogenerative issues, Lyme disease, multiple sclerosis, type-2 diabetes, depression, anxiety, and paranoia.

One example of a device that mimics altitude training is the 02 Trainer created by Bas Rutten, which can be used during

---

42 Angela Navarrete-Opazo and Gordon S. Mitchell, "Therapeutic Potential of Intermittent Hypoxia: A Matter of Dose," *American Physiological Society*, September 17, 2014, 307(10): 1181-97.

breathwork or athletic training to reduce oxygen flow and stimulate the lungs and diaphragm to work harder to pull in oxygen—resulting in increased cardiovascular performance and reduced stress.

Hyperbaric and Hypobaric Oxygen Chambers

Another advanced method to bring more oxygen to the body is to use a hyperbaric oxygen chamber, which is a super-oxygenated tank. A hyperbaric oxygen chamber has greater-than-normal barometric pressure, similar to what you'd experience scuba diving. The increased oxygen stimulates the healing process, and the pressure helps oxygen go deep into your tissues and cells.

Hyperbaric oxygen chambers are found at medical facilities and hospitals, where they're used to relieve pain and promote healing by hyperoxygenating the body, stimulating stem cells and regulating the sympathetic and parasympathetic nervous systems. They're used to help heal, speed up recovery, and/or improve brain damage, neurodegeneration, cancers, autism, cerebral palsy, trauma, infections that cause tissue death, anemia, burns, radiation injury, and a variety of other illnesses. They also help the detoxification process.[43] They're also used to reduce recovery and healing time for athletes. Basically, increasing oxygen to the body and cells improves the function of every system.

If you decide to use one, the medical staff will take you through the proper procedures. Sessions can be expensive—around $125 up to $250 per person for an hour. Some

---

43 "Hyperbaric Oxygen Therapy," *Mayo Clinic*, 2019.

facilities will take insurance, depending on your plan. Often, a hyperbaric chamber at a hospital will be reserved for a specific use, for example treating cancer or burns, and you may need to seek out a privatized hyperbaric oxygen chamber for other uses. Private tanks are typically available in every major city.

CVAC MACHINES

While a hyperbaric oxygen chamber can be like taking a dive down into a pressurized environment, a hypobaric chamber is like altitude training that simulates a lower-oxygen environment. The benefit of this kind of training is that it helps the body learn to utilize oxygen more efficiently. One specific type of hypobaric oxygen chamber is the CVAC, which stands for Cyclic Variations in Adaptive Conditioning. A CVAC machine cycles quickly from a high simulated elevation to a low one, rapidly and consistently. CVAC machines have shown to help increase the number of mitochondria (the powerhouses of cells) as well as increase their size.

In short, a CVAC machine can help build both aerobic and anaerobic capacity of the cells, just by sitting in a chamber. By raising and lowering the atmospheric pressure, the chamber creates a pumping effect on your vascular, lymphatic, and even glymphatic systems—the last of which stimulates and detoxes the glial cells in the brain.

CVAC machines are growing in popularity, but there are still only around eighty-five centers across the world that have them. As a result, they're fairly expensive.

I've also combined using the hyperbaric and hypobaric

oxygen chambers with deep breathing—a process which I don't recommend to anyone who is not already an experienced practitioner of the breathwork and familiar with the use of these chambers. Hyperbaric oxygen chamber do come with some risks, so always make sure it is right for you. The staff at the medical facilities I frequented told me that deep breathing in the hyperbaric chamber would not deepen the effect of the chamber, but as I've said, I go by my own experience. They also told me not to hold my breath because of the pressure, but as with many pioneers, I had to go where no man had gone before (at least that I knew of).

I decided to try it little by little, breathing in deeply through my nose and out through my mouth during one session, or I would mix breathing patterns. As I sat in the hyperbaric chamber for an hour, and I felt a more intense healing effect in my brain. I could quite literally feel the healing happening faster. I could also feel the different effects depending on how I breathed. If I breathed through the nose, I would feel more effects in my prefrontal cortex. I noticed afterward that I had more clarity. After a few sessions like this, my brain started to come back from the deep state of illness and confusion I'd been experiencing over the course of being sick. My memory was better, colors were brighter, and I was happier and less depressed.

While as when I went to the hypobaric oxygen chamber at the place called Recover NYC and was practicing and testing out breathwork and breath retention inside the chamber, I found out that one of the owners did the same thing as a hack or enhancement of what was already happening in the chamber. I also was told by his business partner that this owner got in incredibly great shape, both aerobically and anaerobically, just from the chamber alone.

Slowly, one step at a time, I began to experiment with breath holds on the inhale and exhale, and I continued to feel better and better. Some sessions in the hyperbaric oxygen chamber, I actually felt like I was on ecstasy—I had tingling sensations in my body, I was buzzing with energy, and I felt intense euphoria. All of these, I recognized, were signs of high blood oxygen levels, but they also signaled much deeper healing.

Like any practice, I watched my body's responses and expanded my experiments little by little. The key, should you want to try similar experiments, is to pay attention to how your body is responding and adapting, and try new methods in small doses to see what works for you.

OZONE THERAPY

Ozone therapy is another way to improve the body's intake of oxygen as well as activate the immune system. I did ozone therapy at a few places in a few ways and they all have their benefits.

- Blood infused: The staff drew my blood, and then added the odorless gas that has oxygen atoms in it to my blood and shook it around. I could see the color of the blood change from a dark red to a bright red, and then they put it back into the body through an IV.
- Saline infused: This method is done through IV and uses smaller particles; for me, this was a good treatment to target the brain.
- Direct injection: I had ozone injected directly into an area where I was experiencing active Lyme symptoms.
- Ozone enema: This is done rectally, and it is great for people with intestinal or cervical issues.

Ozone is used to help kill viruses and cancer cells; it helps with arthritis and infected wounds, and aids in circulatory issues.

Apparently, Ten Pass Ozone Therapy is an even more advanced version, which is the equivalent to ten hyperbaric treatments. Clinical expert Dr. Howard Robins has administered ozone therapy for over twenty-four years and spoke of the effects: "Ozone acts like a super antioxidant and is super detoxifier that selectively, like a claw or glue, attaches to and eliminates viruses, fungus, yeast, mold, as well as every form of bacteria, toxic metal, and pathogen from the body."[44]

According to Dr. Robins, since 1990 over 45,000 physicians have used ozone therapy to treat herpes, shingles, multiple sclerosis, Lyme disease, rheumatoid arthritis, hepatitis B and C, HPV, diabetic ulcers, peripheral neuropathy, candidiasis, fibromyalgia, chronic fatigue, macular degeneration, glaucoma, and even AIDS.

Oxygen also potentiates other substances, so people who are deficient in nutrients can do ozone therapy alongside an IV of vitamin C or NAD+ and increase the results because the uptake of the nutrients is better with more oxygen. (More on those supplements in the appendix.)

MEDITATION ON ICE

The second component of the Wim Hof Method is to combine the breathing technique with cold exposure.

---

44   Howard Robins, "Ozone: The Miracle Medicine," *Natural Awakenings*, 2018.

To begin training yourself for cold exposure, it is recommended to adapt the body through a twenty-day challenge: take a cold shower every day and gradually increase the time you spend in the cold. The first day, you can begin with just a twenty-second cold shower. Every day, you increase the length of time by ten to fifteen seconds, so that the time you spend gets longer and longer.

Bart Scholtissen, one of the instructors for the Wim Hof Masters Course, has a PhD in neuroscience; when he discovered the Wim Hof Method, he was burned out from his job and didn't know what to do with his life. He ended up becoming a Wim Hof instructor. He began his practice with the twenty-day cold shower challenge, and he described how, after he'd worked himself up to a two-minute shower, he stepped out on the sixth day and all of a sudden, he realized his body was warm. He wondered what the hell was going on—he'd just stepped out of intense cold; how could he be feeling warm? That's when the power of this technique hit him. The body's natural internal regulation mechanisms had turned on, and as a neuroscientist he needed to find out more—which led him to on the path to becoming an instructor trainer.

"I stopped fighting the cold," Scholtissen told me in an interview. "In Western society, when we meet stress, we fight, because that is what we've learned to do. I finally just accepted the fact that it was cold—I accepted the stressor at hand—and then I let my body do what it's supposed to do: warm up. And it did. This beautiful biological mechanism hasn't evolved out of us."[45]

---

45   Bart Scholtissen, in conversation with the author, May 22, 2019.

As Scholtissen learned the Wim Hof breathing techniques, he realized he could also regulate other systems of his body, such as the dopamine in his brain. Over time, he was able to recover from the burnout he'd been experiencing.

If you learn anything from this book, this is perhaps one of the most important lessons: the practice of acceptance is powerful tool. What you resist persists and when you resist the cold, the more painful it is. When you accept something you can't change, it no longer has power over you.

One of the best ways to start a cold exposure practice is just the way Scholtissen started, by gradually increasing the length of time in a cold shower. Like with the breathing techniques, it's important to pay attention to your body's response and not push yourself further than your body wants to go. Never force anything. Everyone's tolerance and capacity are different. I was once on a Wim Hof retreat where I watched a Canadian participant swim in freezing cold water for twenty minutes, and he felt fine the entire time. Meanwhile, all the skinny guys with low body fat were struggling after fifteen minutes in the river. The more you gradually increase your exposure to the elements, the more you can train your nervous system, and the more fit you become.

GRADUATING TO ICE

Once you've trained your system with the twenty-day cold shower challenge, you can expand your practice by working with ice baths.

The sequence of the method is to use the deep fast breaths described earlier, for a few rounds of thirty to fifty breaths with retention holds, and then enter the ice bath. The breathing technique hyperoxygenates and heats the body, releases natural analgesics, making the ice bath easier. The ice bath cools the body, contracts blood vessels, and charges the cells. This heating and cooling action can be used as a pump to expand and contract the blood vessels and lymphatic system.

THE LYMPHATIC SYSTEM

The lymphatic system is an important part of the vascular and immune system. It is a network of vessels, ducts, nodes, tissues, and organs that drain lymph fluid from your tissues into the blood toward the heart. The lymphatic system has multiple functions, including transporting fat and fatty acids from the digestive system, as well as carrying white blood cells to the bones. It plays a pivotal role in clearing wastes from the body.

Like the plumbing system in a house, it's important to keep your lymph flowing, and flowing nicely, for optimal health. If excess waste is dumped into a plumbing system, it gets clogged. In your system, excess toxins, lack of movement, and lack of hydration all slow down the lymphatic system, manifesting in a multitude of ailments, from fatigue and swollen glands to brain fog and chronic sickness.

Here are some proven methods to keep the lymphatic system moving:
- Exercise, yoga, and chi gong
- Deep breathing, and laughing (which activates the diaphragm to help pump the lymphatic system)

- Staying hydrated (particularly with lemon or lime water)
- Rebounding (shaking or jumping, such as on a trampoline, to cause stimulation)
- Dry brushing (taking a dry brush with course bristles and brush the skin towards the heart)
- Massage
- Enzymes, especially from raw food and juices

"PUSH-UPS" FOR THE VASCULAR SYSTEM

The Wim Hof Method trains the eighty thousand miles of your cardiovascular system, even down to the tiny little capillaries in your fingers. For someone who often has cold hands and feet, ice can actually be a great way to train better blood flow and stimulate the natural body heating system. When you're in the ice bath, blood flow naturally restricts as the blood vessels contract to keep the heat in. When you get out and warm your body back up, the blood vessels will actually open up more to get the heat out.

This *vasoconstriction* (contraction) and *vasodilation* (expansion) of the blood vessels can break up the hardening of arteries (called *arterial sclerosis*) and increase the flexibility of your blood vessels. Increased flexibility in the blood vessels gives your circulatory system a larger capacity, as the blood vessels are able to carry more oxygen, nutrients, and hormones to all areas of the body, while carrying more wastes out. This process is like strength training for your cardiovascular system and the cells, because these tiny structures are doing push-ups with each constriction and dilation.

But the greater benefit of practice, in my opinion, is that an ice bath facilitates training your mind—and mindset is the key to true health.

COLD EXPOSURE TRAINS YOUR BRAIN

When you step into an ice bath, your system goes into extreme fight or flight. As soon as the water hits your skin, pain receptors fire and send signals straight to the reptilian, survivalist part of the brain. Your brain tells you, "You're going to die, get out!" That sympathetic stimulation elicits pure reaction if we are not prepared with the right mindset.

By provoking a sympathetic response, you can practice overriding your body's reaction with a cool and controlled response. It's difficult to think in an ice bath; the analytical mind shuts down. You're no longer in the future, or the past—you are in the present. Focus on the breath and accept the cold as a friendly tool to make you healthier, happier, and stronger. The mindfulness practice that is developed in the ice bath is one of the most valuable benefits because you are training your body and mind to deal, cope with, and accept discomfort. Through training with cold exposure, stressful situations in life no longer seem as stressful. It builds character and mental strength.

As Bruce Lee famously said, "Do not pray for an easy life; pray for the strength to endure a difficult one. Don't ask for an easier life; ask for a stronger body and mind so that challenges become easier." This practice is ultimately about letting go; it's about surrendering and acceptance. I promise that the benefits far outweigh the short period of discomfort.

UNDERSTANDING ADAPTATION

When you begin a new practice of any kind, whether it's a breathing technique or working yourself up to sitting in ice baths, it's important to take small steps and see how your body responds. The purpose of these practices is to create adaptation in your body, not to stress your system by doing too much too soon.

Adaptation is successful when you're presented with the right amount of challenge or stress, and your body has the resources to strengthen and grow in response to that challenge. Too much, and you over train—you can create damage to your system, and your body is taxed from having to repair too much at once. This "sweet spot" of adaptation has two terms I would like you to know and understand: *hormesis* and General Adaption Syndrome (GAS).

HORMESIS AND GENERAL ADAPTATION SYNDROME

In 1888, Hugo Schulz was experimenting on a yeast culture and he noticed something interesting. When he sprayed pesticides over the yeast, they would usually die in large doses. But if he sprayed a small amount of pesticide on the culture, the yeast would grow. Given just the right amount of environmental or toxic stress, Schultz realized, an organism can become stronger and have a beneficial adaptation effect on the cells or the organism that would normally be damaging at higher doses. This "sweet spot" of the right amount of stress is called *hormesis*.

Similarly, when we encounter the right amount of stress in our bodies, we can adapt and grow stronger. The cold exposure from an ice bath, for example, can cause the cardiovascular and nervous systems to get stronger, but the medicine is in the dosage. If we stay too long in an ice bath, we can become hypothermic; it's only through the right amount of exposure that we experience the benefits.

When we experience stress, the body responds with physiological changes that are known as *general adaptation syndrome* (GAS).

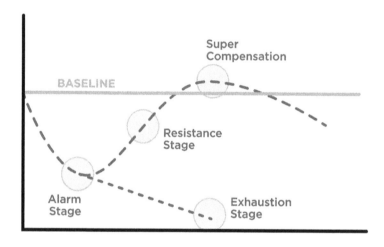

GAS is a three-stage process that was observed and discovered by Hans Seyle at McGill University. Hans was a medical doctor and researcher and observed the series of physiological changes in rats that turned out to be a typical response to stress. The three stages are alarm, resistant, and exhaustive.

Alarm Stage

The alarm state is the initial phase that your body experiences under stress or threat (the flight or fight response). The sympathetic nervous system kicks in and your body prepares to run or fight to be free of the threat. If you have ever done an ice bath or encountered any situation that triggered an alarm state, then you are probably familiar with this.

After the alarm state passes, the body enters the resistant phase: it begins to repair and recover from the threat. Cortisol levels begin to decline, and heart rate and blood pressure move back toward homeostasis. Even though the body is recovering, it can remain on high alert for a period of time depending on the dosage of stress or threat.

Resistant Stage

Stress can continue for long periods of time and the body can remain in the high-alert condition if the threat has been removed. The body will learn to adapt to this level of stress and will go through physiological changes that you may not necessarily be consciously aware of. You may think that you are managing well, but on a physiological level a different story is being told: your blood pressure still remains high, stress hormones are still releasing. The length of the resistant stage depends on the strength and resilience of the organism.

Exhaustive Stage

Next is the exhaustive stage, which is characterized by the signs and symptoms of over-training or too much acute or chronic stress. If we're exposed to prolonged chronic stress, that stress can deplete the body on almost every level—physically, mentally, and emotionally—and can lead to complete burnout as well as a compromised immune system. This is where dis-ease can begin. Signs of the exhaustion stage include depression, anxiety, elevated resting heart rate, severe fatigue, and a low ability to handle stress. I know all three of these stages all too well as I have dealt with them in both training and illnesses myself, and I've been trained to recognize them in others as a certified strength and conditioning specialist.

Recovery

We can use the right amount of stress to our benefit to stimulate GAS. To keep those gains, it's crucial to take time to recover: go home, eat, sleep, and drink water. As your body recovers, it adapts, creating a greater capacity for when the stress might reoccur. This "new normal" is called *supercompensation.*

Our bodies are capable of taking on way more than we think is possible—so long as we get one small dose at a time. As we take on new practices or stress—whether it's breathwork or an ice bath, exercise, or even the stress of a business—it's best to increase the stimulus gradually and watch how the body reacts; that is how someone becomes a master at anything. By listening to our bodies, we can find the "sweet spots" that provide beneficial outcomes making us stronger, building resilience, and speeding up recovery.

LEARNING FROM EXPERIENCE

The first real ice bath I ever did was five minutes long. When I trained with Wim in Spain, we did a fifteen-minute river immersion one day and a fifteen-minute ice bath the next day, and then I took a break for a while. Since it was my first time, I needed a little time to recover. For a while, I only took short cold showers, and then went back to progressively longer ice baths: first five minutes, then seven, then ten minutes, then twelve and fifteen and so on.

Eventually, I worked my way up to a twenty-minute ice bath. Here's where I went wrong. Any time you're trying to gradually adapt your body to a new level, you should only change one variable at a time and also stick to a training program. For example, extending the length of time in the ice bath and lowering the temperature would be two variables changed at once. I had increased the normal ice bath temperature I was adapted to—but I didn't stick to my plan of twenty minutes. That's where I went wrong.

I sank into the freezing water and my brain and my body screamed at me to get out (alarm state). I was able to focus and calm myself down (resistant state), and I sat for a long time feeling okay. I looked at the clock: I'd been in for fifteen minutes. *Only five minutes to go,* I thought. Each slow minute ticked by, and I was actually feeling really good, so I decided to stay in longer; in all, I stayed in the ice bath for twenty-five minutes.

At first, I felt okay. But here is the thing: The ice bath isn't always the hardest part. The most challenging part can be five minutes after the ice bath, while the body is warming back up.

I began to shake uncontrollably. People who practice in ice baths or get stuck in freezing weather too long know this as the "after drop." The "after drop" occurs when cold blood from the arms and legs returns to the core. When the body is not adapted, the temperature is too cold or the duration is too long, the temperature of the blood returning from the extremities is too low, and can actually cause the core temperature to drop even more. That's what happened to me: I was on the verge of mild hypothermia. I was having a serious challenge trying to warm up naturally. I went into a hot shower and stayed there for half an hour—I just couldn't warm up. I'd missed the sweet spot of adaptation. Instead, all my energy was going into damage control.

I didn't even want to *look* at an ice bath for three or four weeks after that. When you're no longer interested in a practice you were drawn to, that's a blatant sign of overtraining or hitting that exhaustive state. When I finally returned to sit in an ice bath, I felt just as much nervousness and fear as I had when I was encountering it for the first time. Like any exercise, it's important to take breathwork and ice bath practices seriously and in a slow progression so that you can feel the benefits of it and keep yourself from overtraining.

THE HACKS

Accessible Methods
- Buteyko Breathing
- Box Breathing
- Altitude Training
- Twenty-Day Cold Shower Challenge

Advanced Methods
- Ice Baths
- Intermittent Hypoxia Therapy
- Hyperbaric Oxygen Chambers
- Hypobaric Oxygen Chambers (CVAC)
- Ozone Therapy

Combining the Hacks

- Set an intention before doing breathwork and per-form the Liquid Light meditation directly afterward. I have seen many powerful transformations and trauma releases in people who practice this combination.
- For increased results, try breathwork before, after, or during PEMF therapy or a session in a hyperbaric oxygen chamber.

Things to Consider Avoiding

- Avoid chest breathing, or through your mouth all day. Pay attention to the quality of your breath through-out the day. You can set a timer to remind yourself to take time for conscious breathing. Two to three times a day, take fuller, deeper, controlled breaths through your nose and down into your belly. I recommend morning, afternoon, and before bed to my clients. It can take as little as one minute to dramatically alter your physiology and mindset for the better by simply taking ten to twenty deep breaths.

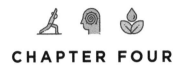

CHAPTER FOUR

MOVEMENT MATTERS

We often approach a new physical training program because we're seeking a specific physical change, but movement is crucial to all of our body's systems. Every cell of your body is essentially a mini "you," and in the same way that you need nutrients and oxygen and blood flow, each cell in your body does, too.

Each cell has its own nervous system, excretory system, digestive system, elimination system, and lymphatic system. Cells get these needs met through movement: literally the movement of nutrients, oxygen, carbon dioxide, and other substances in and out of each cell. When the cells don't have movement, they're not able to exchange nutrients and balance themselves—and that's when we see disease and discomfort in our bodies.

If we are not moving a lot and often, then we are inviting mental, physical, and emotional issues into our lives. Movement is medicine, and the type of movement needed varies per the situation. If you need healing, a lighter, easier, and energy-producing movement is best, rather than a strenuous exercise that depletes your energy and stimulates the sympathetic nervous system.

MOVEMENT REDUCES INFLAMMATION

Being inactive increases your risk for numerous diseases, including type II diabetes, cardiovascular disease, chronic obstructive pulmonary disease, colon cancer, breast cancer, dementia, and depression.[46] Each of these conditions is connected to inflammation. Exercise causes levels of cytokines—inflammatory markers in the blood—to go down.[47]

In the case of depression, which I used to suffer from, the brain is in low-grade inflammation. I was diagnosed with depression as a teenager, but as I decreased my overall levels of inflammation through releasing emotions, proper nutrition, and removing alcohol along my healing journey, my depression went away. By reducing inflammation across the whole system, we can resolve illness.

Conversely, lack of activity stimulates the network of inflammatory pathways, and it leads to visceral fat. A cascading effect results: as people gain weight and become more sedentary, they tend to eat more poorly and store more toxins. Chronic inflammation can set in and promote the development of insulin resistance and the hardening of arteries (and arterial sclerosis, the disease that results from hardened arteries, is the number-one silent killer).[48] Neurodegeneration results from inactivity, and certain cancers grow under inflamed conditions. All of this results from physical inactivity.

---

46 M. Gleeson, et al, "The Anti-Inflammatory Effects of Exercise: Mechanisms and Implications for the Prevention and Treatment of Disease," *Nature Reviews Immunology*, August 5, 2011, 11(9): 607-15.

47 Kyle L. Timmerman, et al, "Exercise Training-Induced Lowering of Inflammatory (CD14+CD16+) Monocytes: A Role in the Anti-Inflammatory Influence of Exercise?" *Journal of Leukocyte Biology*, July 29, 2008.

48 "Heart Disease Facts," *Centers for Disease Control and Prevention.*

The inverse, though, is that as people exercise adaptively, they protect against chronic inflammation and its associated diseases. Fat mass goes down, along with visceral fat. Anti-inflammatory pathways are stimulated, and inflammation pathways are deactivated with every bout of exercise.

A study found that compared with a sedentary state, moderate exercise is associated with reduced incidences of infection.[49] But as we've described before, it's important to not do too much too fast. The same study found that elite athletes who do frequent, intense training are actually more susceptible to infection.

Exercise also has an effect on our *microbiome.* This diverse culture of bacteria in our gut helps us digest food, secretes neurochemicals, and plays a major role in our immune system. One study described how overtraining damages the microbiome and the cell lining of the intestines and complicates the inflammatory response.[50] That's what happened to me: my intense, constant training resulted in inflammation, mixed with gut-damaging medication and ultimately infection and disease. The main takeaway, however, is that movement and exercise are directly connected to preventing disease and reducing inflammation. We need it in the right amounts and degrees of intensity that feel good to us.

49   Stephen A. Martin, Brandt D. Pence, and Jeffrey A. Woods, "Exercise and Respiratory Tract Viral Infections," *Exercise and Sport Sciences Reviews,*" October 2009, 37(4): 157-164.

50   Allison Clark and Nuria Mach, "Exercise-Induced Stress Behavior, Gut-Microbiota-Brain Axis and Diet: A Systematic Review for Athletes," *Journal of the International Society of Sports Nutrition,* November 24, 2016.

GOOD INFLAMMATION AND BAD INFLAMMATION

Soreness—which is actually inflammation—is a normal result of working out. In chapter two, we discussed how chronic inflammation results in a variety of illnesses and dis-ease. Intermittent inflammation, such as muscle soreness, is a normal part of the body's repair mechanisms. If you work out regularly and go through frequent soreness and recovery, your body will adapt, and get faster and more efficient at repairing itself. In fact, with regular training, I consistently see our clients recover from injury, surgery, or childbirth dramatically faster.[51]

An incredible illustration of this is the story of our client Nancy, who was diagnosed with cancer. She had already been training at our facility for a long period of time, and when doctors caught the cancer in her lungs, they realized she would need surgery. Nancy was older, and her doctors were impressed that she felt in good health despite how the cancer had progressed. They attributed her relative health to her level of fitness. During the lung surgery, they had to put a temporary tube in her lungs. When they went to remove the tube, her skin and tissues had healed so quickly around it that the tube was stuck. The doctor got it out, after a bit more pain than was typical, but he remarked that he'd never seen someone's skin heal so fast around the tube.

The increased oxygen we get in our bodies from exercise is a huge part of speedier recovery. Like we talked about in the previous chapter, breathwork, hyperbaric oxygen chambers, and ozone therapy are excellent recovery tools because of how much these methods can increase oxygen levels in the body.

---

51 Thomas J. Hoogeboom, et al, "Merits of Exercise Therapy Before and After Major Surgery," *Current Opinions in Anaesthesiology*, April 2014, 27(2): 161-166.

Oxygen assists in the changeover of cells: it helps clear out dead cells and set the stage for new cells to thrive. Movement and oxygen together stimulate the healing process.

So how do you know whether you're creating good inflammation or bad inflammation? It has to do with how long the inflammation lasts. When our body is in a constant state of inflammation, it never fully recovers; it can't clear out damaged tissues or rejuvenate cells. The general rule of thumb is that if you have muscle soreness for longer than seventy-two hours, that's a good indicator you've pushed your body too hard. If you have chronic inflammation in the body for longer than that, you want to make sure you put out the fire ASAP using some of the techniques in this book. Find the root cause of your inflammation so it doesn't resurface.

MOVING THROUGH INJURY

Movement isn't just something we need when we're feeling well and healthy; it's still necessary for our bodies when we're injured. When we have someone come into our training facility with one arm in a sling, we look to what else they can move: their good shoulder and their legs. Keeping the rest of the body moving will increase the rate of recovery to the injured area, and it can actually prevent atrophy in the muscles of the injured limb.

When someone does a shoulder press with their good arm, there is a diffusion of motor impulses from the spinal pathway to the injured limb.[52] By completing shoulder presses with the good arm, it helps maintain muscle mass on the injured side even though it's not being exercised. Studies have shown close to 30 percent transference of what is being lifted on the opposite arm gets activated in the unused arm.[53]

The same benefits of exercise, including increased oxygen, blood flow and nutrients, will stimulate the healing process and help the injury recover faster. Keep in mind that when the body is injured, there's inflammation protecting the area and helping it heal. In an injured state, overtraining and pushing too hard can set a person back. You need just enough stimulus to get blood flowing. At times when we're injured, just doing visualization and breathwork alone can be powerful. In fact, scientists have proven simply imagining exercises can prevent muscle atrophy, make you stronger, and tone your muscles (but save that for the worst-case scenario, and move your body frequently).[54] Combined with light movement, the benefits of breathwork are exponentially greater.

STABILIZING BLOOD SUGAR

The more you can stabilize your blood sugar, the longer you will live. Working out is a great way to stabilize blood sugar

52   Jonathan Farthing and Justin Andrushko, "Exercising Healthy Limb May Fight Atrophy in Broken One," *CNN Health*, October 9, 2018.

53   Robin R. Hlavacek, "The Effecgts of Contralateral Limb Strength Training on Muscle Atrophy in an Immobilized Upper Extremity," *Masters Thesis*, 1996.

54   Charlene Adams, "Scientists Discover Just Imagining Exercising Can Make You Stronger, Tone Your Muscles, and Delay or Stop Muscle Atrophy," *Daily Mail*, December 24, 2014.

levels. As muscles work, they require more glucose for fuel. If you train before you eat, you can reduce blood sugar spikes because your muscles will consume the sugars from your food. Because sugars are being quickly absorbed by muscles, they don't hang out in the blood stream or get stored as fat. You can actually lower your blood sugar level up to twenty-four hours after a workout.[55] This is why athletes can tend to eat whatever they want: they are so active that their muscles are constantly consuming sugars, and as a result their blood sugar levels stay lower.

At our training facility, a lot of clients come in with prediabetes, which means they've sustained a high level of blood sugar for a long period of time. Doctors give their patients medications for prediabetes, but it's actually a metabolic disease, which means it's a condition that can be reversed through exercise and diet.

In fact, if you have prediabetes or type-II diabetes, the number one thing you can do to boost your health right away is to begin an exercise program. You can also reduce the number of times your blood sugar spikes by lowering your carb intake. But simply increasing the amount of movement in your day will stabilize your blood sugar and insulin levels. I just received yet another report of a client no longer having prediabetes after a couple years of training at my facility.

---

55 "Blood Sugar and Exercise," *American Diabetes Association*, 2019.

A MOVEMENT HACK FOR DINING OUT

It's common that when people go out to eat, they often decide to indulge in a food that they know will spike their blood sugar more than usual. Knowing that movement creates more demand for sugar for the muscles, you can use this process to your advantage.

Before heading out to a restaurant, or even while you are at the restaurant, I have even heard Ben Greenfield, a famous biohacker, say that he will go to the bathroom and do a quick round of movement: a minute or two of fast squats or pushups (you can do pushups with your hands on the counter to give yourself an easier incline) will help mitigate the blood sugar spike you'll later get from your meal.

COMING BACK STRONGER

In addition to reducing inflammation and stabilizing blood sugar, movement creates stress on the body that then, during recovery, allows the body to heal and build back stronger. A good example of this is how exercise strengthens bones.

Bones can become more brittle from lack of movement, from too much stress on the bones, or from lack of nutrients. Your blood has to maintain a certain level of minerals, and if the body is not getting what it needs through diet, it will leach what it needs from other areas—and your bones are the perfect source for key minerals the whole body needs, including magnesium and Vitamins D, C, and K (which is found in leafy greens and limes). I recommend a good core minerals supplement, like ReMyte by Dr. Carol Dean, to ensure the body has what it needs to maintain strong bones. Exercise is another critical component of bone health.

As you move, particularly with strenuous exercise, your network of osteocytes (bone cells) cracks slightly. Once you go home and eat, sleep, and recover, your body repairs these cracks and builds your bones back stronger. Typically, it takes a certain amount of stress on the bones to create adaptation, which is why progressive programing and training is important, meaning that as you get stronger and in better shape you use heavier weights or increase intensity.

In our Back Pain Relief4Life program, we've had clients come in with osteoporosis of the spine, whose doctors have told them the damage was irreversible. But after doing the Back Pain Relief4Life program combined with a year or two of strength training, these clients go back to their doctors and find that their conditions have reversed from osteoporosis to osteopenia (meaning their bones have gotten denser). They're able to lift extremely heavy weight and their back pain has disappeared. And eventually, they no longer have osteopenia. We have seen this progression occur many times, and it's a testament to how the body can heal itself when given what it needs.

You have the power at any time, at any age, to repair, rebuild, and strengthen your body. Don't let anyone tell you differently.

LUBRICATING JOINTS

Movement stimulates production of synovial fluid that lubricates the joints. Again, we see a clear illustration of these effects in our Back Pain Relief4Life program. One of the exercises we do (the Chair Pull, described later in this chapter) causes compression in the low back. This often feels counter-intuitive to people: they wonder how compression could decrease their low back pain. The answer is that the joints, nerves, muscles, and tissues need to be stimulated in order to create a response. That's why bed rest is absolutely terrible for back pain. Instead, we need movement around all those joints to get synovial fluid, nutrients, blood flow, and oxygen back to those areas to heal. The Chair Pull will literally activate the muscles and nerves in the lower spine, squeeze blood out and draw new fresh blood in, as well as activate synovial fluid to provide more nutrients.

The same is true for every joint in the body. The spine is, essentially, just a series of joints stacked on top of one another, and the stimulation, movement, and compression that works to heal the spine also works to heal shoulders, hips, knees, and every other joint.

HOW EXERCISE BENEFITS YOUR BRAIN

Exercise creates positive effects on cognitive performance,[56] and it stimulates the release of a variety of positive neurochemicals into the brain. We release serotonin, the happy chemical, and endorphins, which are our body's natural painkillers, as well as adrenaline that boosts our performance, among other chemicals.[57] When we get stimulation in the right amount—not too hard or too fast too soon—in many instances we can use exercise as medication for depression or

---

56   Koji Kashihara, et al, "Positive Effects of Acute and Moderate Physical Exercise on Cognition," *Journal of Physiological Anthropology*, 2009, 28(4): 155-164.

57   Simon N. Young, "How to Increase Serotonin in the Human Brain Without Drugs," *Journal of Psychiatry and Neuroscience*, November 2001, 32(6): 394-399.

anxiety. It's also possible to get addicted to exercise and the adrenaline and endorphins that are released. For the brain, as well as for the rest of the body, exercise in moderation and in balance with recovery is ideal.

A study examining the effect of exercise on depression in mice showed that consistent stress can cause brain damage and neurodegeneration.[58] Specifically, the study focused on the hippocampus, which is the part of the brain associated with depressive behavior. Under stress, the brain creates fewer blood vessels to supply the hippocampus, and that decreased density of blood vessels—and therefore decreased blood flow—results in depression-like behavior. But with increased exercise, you stimulate more blood flow and oxygen to the brain, open up the blood vessels, and increase the nutrient and neurochemical exchange—therefore creating an antidepressant effect. Cognitive function and mental focus go up as a result of exercise.

THE BACK PAIN RELIEF4LIFE PROGRAM

I grew up playing all almost every sport we had an opportunity to play, but when I was about eleven, I fell in love with basketball, and that became my main focus. At fifteen, I tried out for the Connecticut Starter Amateur Athletic Union team and was happy to be selected. We were playing in a tournament when I jumped up to block a pass and had my feet taken out from under me. I landed directly on my spine. I never went to the hospital to check it out; I just dealt with the pain. A year later, the same thing happened while jumping for a rebound, breaking part of my vertebrae.

---

58   T. Kiuchi, H. Lee, and T. Mikami, "Regular Exercise Cures Depression-Like Behavior Via VEGF-Flk-1 Signaling in Chronically Stressed Mice," *Neuroscience*, April 5, 2012, 207: 208–217.

I thought I was doomed to live with back pain for the rest of my life. I tried massage therapy, pain medicine, acupuncture, ultrasound, electric stimulation, the sheets of exercises given to me by physical therapists, yoga, chiropractic, pilates, a stress-relief therapy called alphabiotics and even Kinesis Myofacial Integration, offered at a whopping $125 per session for a minimum of twelve sessions. I was paying cash for that at twenty-four years old while bartending and attending college—but the pain was so severe that I sought to solve it at any expense. Truthfully, I could write a book alone on this subject.

As I entered the health and fitness field, I became a back pain relief expert, helping others eliminate their back pain. I co-created one of the most successful back pain programs in the world and on the internet today. But more importantly, it has helped thousands of people relieve severe and serious back pain. Many times, people come to me as a last resort before surgery and were able to relieve their pain without going under the knife.

More than 80 percent of the population will deal with back pain at one point in their lives.[59] We have a great way to help our clients when they encounter it.

The Back Pain Relief4Life program is a step-by-step system of movements designed to eliminate pain in the simplest and most effective way, naturally. It's often counterintuitive to people who are suffering from debilitating pain to believe that exercises alone can relieve it, but results don't lie: since the release of this program, thousands of people all around

---

59 "Low Back Pain Fact Sheet," *National Institute of Neurological Disorders and Stroke*, 2019.

the world in over one hundred countries have completely eliminated their back pain.

Clients have told me that nothing helped their back pain—including painkillers, steroids, and cortisone injections—but that the back pain program brought them relief from their very first session. "I was skeptical until I tried it," admitted one of my past clients, Dr. Greenwalt. "But I came in hobbling and I left walking." Other clients told me they were able to stop their frequent visits to chiropractors and doctors. A grandmother of five who completed the program described how overjoyed she was to be able to finally bend down and pick up her grandchildren.

All these testimonies, to me, point to the power of movement in healing our bodies, our minds, and our lives.

The program includes eight specific movements that are designed to mobilize the hips, stabilize and decompress the spine, strengthen the core, activate synovial fluid, and bring healing nutrients, blood flow, and oxygen to the lower back and spinal discs.

Most people have very tight hips; sitting at a desk all day makes the hips more stable and less mobile, and the lower back becomes more mobile and less stable—which sets up a recipe for disaster. It should be the opposite: You want to have mobile hips and a stable and strong back and abs.

When people lead sedentary lifestyles, blood flow decreases, and the muscles around the spine lose strength. When people in this compromised state go to pick up something heavy for example, the muscles that help them flex their spine don't properly engage; they hunch as they pick up the heavy object, and all those forces go straight to the lower back. More specifically, due to a lack of energy and strength in the muscles, those forces put strain on the spinal discs. For someone who doesn't have core integrity and stability abound the spine, this movement over time can create micro-trauma, small injuries to the back until one day—*bam!*—a macro trauma like a slipped, bulging, or herniated disc occurs as the back takes strain from poor posture and lack of strength and integrity.

Our posture also creates ripple effects for our mood and our lives. Like many of the issues described in this book, back pain can result when we're disconnected from our natural movement patterns. The exercises in this series connect us back to these primal movements, and they stimulate deep neurological pathways that help improve mood and overall wellbeing.

Practice the following eight exercises three times a week and you will improve mobility, flexibility, core strength, posture, sleep, strength in the back and abs, and a better mind-body connection.

THE EXERCISES

When doing this program, remember that everyone is different. A single set of each exercise may be more than enough for one person on the first day, whereas another person may be able to do three sets at maximal capacity and feel totally fine. Pay attention to your own capacity and adjust the intensity and repetition as needed.

The first four movements start and end in the same position.

Lay supine with your knees bent and feet flat on the floor, about a foot away from your buttocks. Use a small pillow or ball under your head for the correct biomechanical position. Bring your hands by your sides, palms on the floor. Press your back down firmly and engage your abs.

How do you know if your abs are engaged? Here's a simple trick: cough, and feel how your muscles contract. When we cough, the body's natural response is to activate the abs. Connect with that feeling, and create the same engagement in your abs the entire time while doing these exercises. This can take some practice.

KNEE PULL

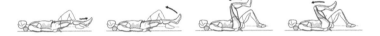

With your spine pressed to the floor and hands pressed down at your sides to engage your nervous system, relax the neck and focus your mind on engaging the abs. Pull your right knee into your chest in a slow, controlled motion until you feel a good stretch in your lower back and feel your abs fully activate. Slowly kick your leg back out, parallel to the floor, and straighten your leg fully. Bring your straight leg as close to the floor as you can without allowing it to touch.

Repeat the knee pull and extension for eight repetitions. With each repetition, increase your range of motion and effort. Then switch to the left side. Do up to three sets, depending on how your body feels. This movement is designed to activate and strengthen the abs and begin to mobilize and stretch tight muscles in the back and prepare the body for the next movements.

KNEE DROP

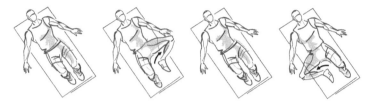

Begin in the same starting position, laying on the floor with knees bent, with a pillow or ball under your head. Open your right knee out to the side, so that you feel your pelvis open, your glutes (buttock muscles) activate, and your inner thigh stretch. Squeeze your right glute to activate the muscle. Bring the knee back upright.

Repeat this motion eight times. Each time you repeat, see if you can increase your range of motion and bring your knee closer to the floor without forcing it. Switch to the left side. Repeat this set three times. This exercise is designed to stretch the inner thigh and fire the glutes.

SINGLE FROG LEG

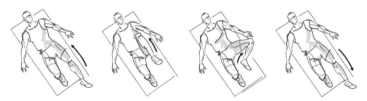

This exercise combines the knee pull and the knee drop with a slight variation. From the starting position, first do a knee pull with your right leg, and then take your right knee out to the side in a half-circle motion, keeping the abs tight and the pelvis and low back in a stable strong position. You want to make sure that your abs are fully activated and you are still pulling your pelvis in while circling the knee out to the side.

Then kick the leg out. Keep the sole of your foot close to the inner thigh, rotating as you go, until the right leg is parallel to the floor. Repeat this sequence eight times, and switch to the left side. Do three sets, or as many as feel good for your back and your body. This is designed to stretch the lower back and activate the glutes and hip rotators. We are reconnecting the mind with these muscles and movements. This is a primal movement pattern that you may not have done since you were a baby.

DOUBLE FROG LEG

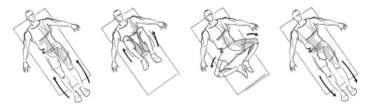

This move is more advanced, and you'll need to have the ability to fully engage your abs and keep your back flat. The double frog leg is just like the single frog leg, but this time you'll move both legs at the same time. It's important to keep your back firmly pressed against the floor, and your palms flat by your sides. Don't extend the legs so far that you lose the engagement of your abs. Maintain control to keep the spine stable and flat on the floor. The idea is to open your legs out as far as you can as you slowly kick the legs forward.

You can also adjust the intensity of this movement to three levels. In level one, instead of extending your legs out parallel to the floor, you can extend them straight up so they're perpendicular. This takes pressure off the abs. When you've established control with that movement, you can try level two: take the legs out to a 45-degree angle. Finally, in level three, you can extend your legs to a hover just above the floor. This exercise activates the lower back muscles, the glutes, the pelvis, the inner thighs, and the hip rotators. Again, if you feel like you need more guidance you can check out our online programs at backpainrelief4life.com.

CHRYSALIS STRETCH

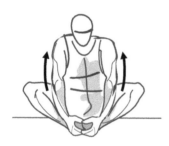 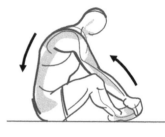

While many people may confuse this with the "butterfly stretch," we call it a chrysalis instead, because this is where transformation occurs. Sit upright, bend your knees, and bring the soles of your feet together with the outside edges of your feet on the floor. Sit up nice and straight, hold your feet, and slowly move your lower back forward. Try not to round your spine so much; although your upper back may round, keep your lower back straight and hinge at the hips. Pull your forehead toward your toes until you feel a stretch in your low back.

Many people have trouble accessing stretch in the low back in this pose because their inner thighs may be too tight. That's why it's important to practice these exercises at least three times a week in order to progress with each session. You can also adjust your feet by moving them forward if you feel your inner thighs stretch too much. You'll feel stretch in the muscles that are tightest for you: hips, glutes, inner thighs, or low back. Hold this for eight to twelve seconds. Repeat for three sets.

SEATED JACK KNIFE

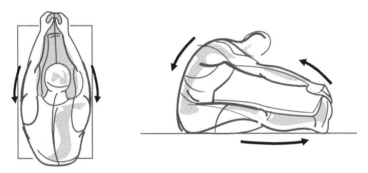

Sit upright and extend your legs straight out in front of you. Press your feet together and bring your ankles as close together as you can. Sit up nice and straight, and then slide your hands down your legs, reaching for your toes. Make sure to initiate the movement by bringing your low back forward, not by rounding in your back. As your flexibility allows, bring your forehead toward your knees, tucking your chin.

Many people feel a stretch in their calves and hamstrings in this pose; in the end, we also want to feel a stretch in the low back. If the hamstrings are super tight, it may take more than a few sessions to feel a stretch in the back. The goal of this is to feel a stretch in the lower back. Some people can get a great assist with a stretching strap. We use our Super Stretching

Strap, which you may be able to get at getrelief4life.com or mybackpaincoach.com if we have them in stock.

BIO CRUNCH

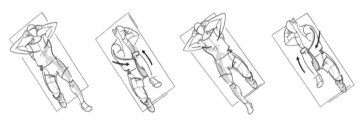

We call this exercise the "bio crunch" because it's the biomechanically correct position to do an ab crunch specific to the obliques, which are important for rotational stability. The main thing is to make sure that you do not rotate the spine. Lay down with your knees bent, feet flat on the floor and about a foot away from your buttocks. Take your right hand gently behind your head. Reach your left arm straight out to the side, with your palm down. Keep the elbow touching the ground at all times. If it comes off while doing the exercise, then you are performing the movement incorrectly.

Bring your right elbow across the body to touch your left knee, right above the midpoint of your belly. If you can't touch them together, that's okay; just try to get them as close as you can by engaging your abs. This exercise targets the oblique muscles that are responsible for rotating your trunk, and it activates muscles that stabilize the spine. Repeat the exercise eight times, and then switch sides. Do three sets.

There are progressive levels to this exercise, and the previous description was level one. For level two, you can begin by extending the left leg out straight, parallel to the floor, without touching the floor. As you cross our right elbow to your left knee, tuck your left knee into your chest. As you release the crunch, extend your left leg straight once more. Repeat the exercise eight times, and switch to the left side, extending the right leg parallel to the floor.

In level three, you can "bicycle" your legs. Begin with both hands behind your head, and bring your legs up at a 90-degree angle. Rotate your trunk and bring your right elbow to your left knee while you extend the right leg, and touch your left elbow to the floor. Come back to center and twist the other way, touching your left elbow to your right knee, and touching your right elbow to the floor. Repeat for three sets of eight repetitions.

CHAIR PULL

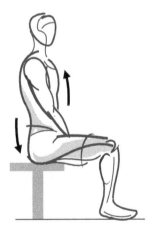 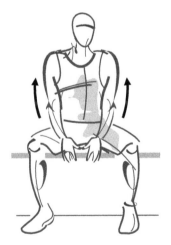

In this final exercise, begin seated on the edge of a chair with your feet flat on the floor. Sit up nice and straight. Separate your legs enough that you can grip the seat of the chair with your hands between your knees. Alternately, you can wrap a strap around the chair and hold the ends of the strap. As you sit up straight, push your buttocks down into the chair and your heels down into the floor, and pull up with your hands. This subtle movement contracts the muscles along your spine, similar to doing a proper deadlift.

This exercise is where a lot of the magic happens, because the spine benefits from engaged compression especially after the specific exercises that were just performed—that's how synovial fluid is activated to lubricate the discs. Additionally, the muscle contraction stimulates blood flow and allows oxygen and nutrients to flow into the low back. This can also help pull discs back into the proper position.

AFTER-EXERCISE CARE

After completing these exercises, for best results, lay down on the floor with your feet propped up on the chair and your knees bent at 90 degrees, keep your back warm (you can wrap it with a sweater or towel) and close your eyes and do a meditation or controlled breathing. Or use the liquid gold meditation with focus on the golden light pouring into the lower back or any area that needs some healing,

As you go through the rest of your day, make sure to drink plenty of water. Pay attention to your posture and notice when you're hunching over or sitting to one side. Try to be conscious of not being in an awkward or uncomfortable position, especially directly after the program. Be conscious of how you're moving and be sure to squat when you pick things up, rather than round your back.

In addition to the instructions here, you can also find videos for this program on the Back Pain Relief4Life website: back-painrelief4life.com. It's even more powerful to work with a person who is certified to execute the Back Pain Relief4Life program; they can help you get more results in a shorter period of time.

THE HACKS

Accessible Methods
- The BackPainRelief4Life Program
- Recovery Training

Advanced Methods
- Working with a quality coach and or trainer to enhance your results

Combining the Hacks
- Do the BackRelief4Life program with breathwork (such as the Wim Hof Method) before the session, and the Liquid Golden Light meditation after the session

Things to Consider Avoiding
- Don't overdo exercise too fast, too hard, or too soon. Use your exercise to help you pay attention to your body and grow a deeper connection with your needs. Always start light and easy, and pay attention to how you feel afterward.

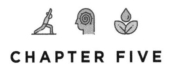

CHAPTER FIVE

FOOD AS MEDICINE

At the time I was profiled in *Men's Health* magazine, I was eating eight to ten thousand calories per day. I was a machine. I was training and eating so much that I didn't have time to truly think about what I was putting in my body. Although I was still health conscious for the most part, I thought I could get away with eating whatever I wanted, or whatever was available.

Miguel Bethelery describes how eating the wrong foods is like putting the wrong type of gas in your car. "We need to give the body what it needs. If you've been putting diesel in your standard gasoline engine, the first thing you need to do is stop and put regular gas in your car. The second thing you need to do is cleanse your engine."[60] The way I had been eating, I didn't understand how much the type of fuel mattered, and I didn't think about what I would be doing to my engine long term. I was only thinking about how to best fuel my energy systems in preparation for the Urbanathlon, based on what I knew at the time.

---

60 Miguel Bethelery, in conversation with the author, January 10, 2019.

It never occurred to me that I might have an issue with grains, that the destruction to my microbiome from antibiotics made digestion even harder. That story of the last pizza happened while I was still trying to figure out what was happening to me, and soon after, I spoke to Peter Osborne, the "gluten guy," who told me he was sure I had an issue with gluten. He told me to eliminate all grains. I then began to remove processed dairy and processed foods. Within a week or two, it was clear what impact these foods had been having on my body. The mental fog I'd been having lifted a little, and I felt clearer. I could focus easier. I had more energy. The difference was like night and day. This quick improvement in my health illustrated clearly to me the impact nutrition has on the body and the mind.

After the health crisis I went through and the healing I've done, I now realize that for me, grains and starches were a bullet being loaded into a gun. The multiple rounds of antibiotics, steroids, and other previous medications like Accutane and antidepressants I'd been given over the course of my life, and all the other junk that had built up in my body were additional bullets. Remember, too, that during my health crisis I'd been diagnosed with Lyme's disease at one point—so tick bites were another bullet. I later learned that the amalgam fillings in my teeth contained heavy metals that added another toxin in my body and another bullet in the gun. At one point I attempted to do a high dose vitamin C healing regimen, but I didn't know at the time that the type of vitamin C matters—I was using a corn-based GMO vitamin C. And when I finally collapsed on the floor of my apartment, my guts twisted in pain, it was as though the trigger on that loaded gun was being pulled again and again.

My body may have been able to heal from each of these factors individually and on its own, but the combination is what ultimately brought me down. Another thing you will notice is that all the factors I mentioned were unnatural and poisonous to the body.

A large part of the problem was diet. When you put foreign or processed substances in your body that need to be processed out, you contribute to your system's load. Though our bodies are designed to eliminate toxins and process sugars and starches, most people get far too much of these substances in their diet, and they can cause our systems to produce and store excess mucus and toxins.

Starches are the primary culprits that produce mucus, and they also increase blood sugar. Essentially, eating sugar causes a spike in insulin to compensate for the rise in blood sugar, and that insulin spike can cause low-grade inflammation. Sugar is also good food for pathogens. This is why many people heal or feel better with low-carb diets.

The herbalist and healer known as Dr. Sebi believed there was only one disease: mucus. Dr. Sebi saw that by using an alkaline diet full of specific fruits, vegetables, and ancient grains, people could clear out mucus and acids from their bodies, which would clear up the environment in their bodies that was allowing disease to manifest and grow.

Building on this idea, Miguel Bethelery says the body is constantly working to eliminate pathogens. In a state of health, the body is able to eliminate these wastes naturally. Disease, however, is "a manifestation of the body trying to cleanse itself, but not being able to finish the job—it is stuck somewhere. Anytime you're fighting disease, you're fighting the body."[61] Dr. Sebi, Dr. Hulda Clarke, Dr. Morse, Irene Grosjean and Miguel Bethelery, as well as many other naturopathic doctors and healers across the globe, have created protocols to support the body's own natural processes of cleansing out toxins and mucus naturally. These healers all knew the body will heal itself. Our job is to give the body what it needs.

As I've mentioned before, each cell in your body is a mini "you." Each cell has a digestive system, a nervous system, and an immune system. Your cells eat what you eat, and they have to clear out the toxins you ingest or come in contact with. When cells are unable to eliminate these wastes, the toxins build up in your body and wreak all types of havoc on the endocrine system and immune system. When your body is sick, it needs to process out the resulting mucus, and when we take medication, it can block that process. Antibiotics can destroy the gut biome that helps to break down our food.

Food can be poison, or it can be medicine: The foods you eat can deliver nutrients that cells need to operate at their best. Since you need constant fuel, food is one of the best ways to heal: certain foods can keep inflammation and blood sugar levels down. By using your intuition, staying connected with your body, and paying attention to how your body responds to your diet, you can use food to heal. You can also use testing to determine which foods work for you and which foods don't, which we go into later in this chapter.

FINDING THE FOODS THAT WORK FOR YOU

Our individual bodies respond differently to different sub-

---

61   Miguel Bethelery, in conversation with the author, January 10, 2019.

stances. For example, one person could get stung once by a bee and go into anaphylactic shock, while another could be stung ten times and see only minimal redness and pain. Food, too, creates different responses in different people. One person's medicine is another person's poison. It all depends on how your individual immune system responds to your diet.

Why would different people have differing reactions to certain foods? Because our ancestry and our origins are adapted to different foods. Our belief system around foods and our genetics and immune system are all different. There is no person in the world with the same makeup as you. The story of the healer Dr. Sebi illustrates this idea.

Dr. Sebi was not a medical doctor; he adopted the name Dr. Sebi as he became a world-famous healer. The story goes something like this: He became sick in his mid-30s and went to a healer who, in the course of talking to Dr. Sebi about diet and food, asked him, "Where are you from?"

Dr. Sebi replied that he was from Honduras.

"What do they eat there?" the healer asked.

"Rice and beans," Dr. Sebi replied.

"And where is your land of origin? Where are your ancestors from?"

"I'm from Africa," Dr. Sebi said.

"Do they eat rice and beans in Africa?"

No, Dr. Sebi realized—this was not a native diet in his heritage. The healer was making the point that Dr. Sebi had been poisoning himself with the food of Central America, which didn't align with where his genetics had come from or what his ancestors had eaten. The healer recommended that Dr. Sebi fast and then cleanse his body with specific herbs and plants. The process of cleansing and changing his diet transformed Dr. Sebi's life.

From that point on, Dr. Sebi learned the process of healing and began to study plants, herbs, and natural medicine. His healing protocol was based on eating alkaline foods, which he proposed would reduce acid in the body and break up mucus.

He developed a specific list of vegetables, fruits, herbal teas, grains, nuts, seeds, and oils that he described as "cell food" to provide the best nutrition on a cellular level. He also advocated for cutting out meat, dairy, most grains and man-made hybrid foods. In my experience, certain unhealthy people can use Dr. Sebi's dietary recommendations to bring themselves back to health, and once a baseline of health is restored, they can often incorporate other foods into their diet. Rather than a strict set of guidelines to follow, I see Dr. Sebi's recommendations as a tool to experiment with. It's important to pay attention to your own experience with different diets and find what works for you.

CONNECTING FOOD TO HOW YOU FEEL

Remember, at the root of disease is disconnection with the body, and someone who is in ill health or not performing at their best may struggle to feel the effects different foods have on them. For example, I was recently talking to a client at our training facility whose mother had gut issues and trouble sleeping. As the client and I talked, she suspected that her mother's issues might be due to the side effects of coffee. She later explained to her mother that cutting out coffee might relieve her issues, but her mother didn't want to try that. If you don't try eliminating potential triggers from your diet, you won't be able to feel which effects result from which foods. Doing an elimination diet is one of the best ways to figure out the triggers. You'll see very basic instructions for how to start an elimination diet later in this chapter.

Our bodies want live, nutrient-dense foods. We evolved to eat fruit directly off trees and vegetables picked directly from the ground. Packaged and processed food is a new phenomenon. Previously, the only way we preserved food was through fermentation, which is beneficial for us because it boosts beneficial bacteria. Fermented food has shown to decrease social anxiety in young adults,[62] and also help with cognitive function.[63] However, fermentation consumption has declined since it is no longer a necessity.

Food gives us energy, and we can think about the effect of food in terms of frequency and vibration: living plants are electric and full of energy, and when we eat fresh, live food, our own energy levels rise. We are electrical beings, so it only makes sense that we eat food that charges our batteries.

On the other hand, certain foods have a depleting effect on

---

62 Matthew R. Hilimire, Jordan E. DeVylder, and Catherine A. Forestell, "Fermented Foods, Neuroticism, and Social Anxiety: An Interaction Model," *Psychiatry Research*, 2015, 228(2): 203.

63 Bhagavathi Sundaram Sivamaruthi, Periyanaina Kesika, and Chaiyavat Chaiyasut, "Impact of Fermented Foods on Human Cognitive Function—A Review of Outcome of Clinical Trials," *Scientia Pharmaceutica*, 2018, 86(2): 22.

our energy, and drain our biobatteries, the cells. Pesticides that are sprayed on conventional crops are an example of this. These chemicals are designed to be destructive to life—to pests—and they are also destructive to the microbiota in our gut biomes. If they kill pests, what do you think they do to your cells?

To better understand why certain foods give us the energy and nutrition we need, and other foods deplete our energy, let's take a closer look at the function of the gut and the microbiota within it.

GAPS IN THE GUT

Our intestines are extremely sensitive, and they are constantly regenerating. The cells of the intestinal lining are turned over faster than almost any other part of the body.[64] The intestinal lining has little tentacle structures called *microvilli* that absorb nutrients from our food. In the tissues of the villi, tiny gaps can be created that allow nutrients to pass through into our bloodstream. When the gut is healthy, this barrier keeps out pathogenic substances and undigested food particles, and absorbs only the elements our bodies need.

Another crucial element to our gut function is the microbiota of our intestines. We have a vast diversity of bacteria in our guts, some of which are beneficial and some of which are harmful. The beneficial bacteria help break down our food, and they also keep the harmful bacteria in check.

In addition to digesting our food, our microbiome triggers

---

64 Anthony Samsel and Stephanie Seneff, "Glyphosate, Pathways to Modern Diseases II: Celiac Sprue and Gluten Intolerance," *Interdisciplinary Toxicology*, 2013, 6(4): 159-184.

neurochemicals that communicate with the brain, stimulate our cravings, help induce sleep, and regulate our moods. In fact, a study by the American Gut Project showed that gut bacteria diversity was linked to mental health conditions such as PTSD, schizophrenia, depression, and bipolar disorder.[65] Serotonin is produced in the gut as a result of our beneficial bacteria. Among other neurochemicals, serotonin has a huge effect on our mood.

When we're not producing enough serotonin, life feels a bit duller. A lack of serotonin can lead to anxiety, depression, panic attacks, insomnia, obesity, fibromyalgia, eating disorders, chronic pain, migraines, alcohol abuse, premenstrual syndrome, irritable bowel syndrome, and negative or obsessive thoughts and behaviors.[66]

When I began my holistic healing journey, my first focus was to heal my gut—and in turn, I learned, I would help heal my brain and improve my outlook and mood. One of the first things I did was made my own raw kefir, which is a fermented dairy product. I remember drinking the kefir, getting super sleepy, falling asleep, and waking up feeling really happy— happier than I had been since getting sick. You will often hear people talk about dairy being the devil, but depending on the person, their genetics and their issue, raw dairy and fermented dairy can have many medicinal benefits; because of the beneficial bacteria in raw dairy, it can heal the gut and help restore diversity to the microbiome.

---

65   Joshua Greenberg, "World's Largest Study on the Human Gut Reveals Connection to These Mental Health Problems," *Real Farmacy*.

66   Stacy Sampson, "Serotonin Deficiency: What We Do and Don't Know," *Healthline*, February 27, 2019.

The more diversity in your gut, the better your immune system is. In an interview with me, Sachin Patel, retired functional doctor and founder of The Living Proof Institute, said you can visualize your digestive system as a sprinkler hose in a garden, with little holes to allow nutrients into your body. Your digestive system runs through you, and technically what's inside the digestive system—the food we eat and the bacteria that inhabit our gut—is outside of you. The gut is "an interface between your inside world and outside world," Patel said. "We want a beautiful garden down there, not a weed lot. What we eat matters, and how well we digest matters."[67] To cultivate a healthy garden, we need to eat healthy, live foods and pay attention to how we feel as we're digesting.

In an interview with Dr. Marisol Tejero, a naturopath, she introduced a term she coined called the "conbiotic." Conbiotics are the con artists of the bacterial world because they set up residence in the gut and compete for space, pushing out the "good guys," or the bacteria that make our B vitamins, serotonin, and other essential neurotransmitters, such as melatonin, which helps induce sleep. Common conbiotics include *candida* (also known as yeast), *C. difficile*, and *E. coli*, and *Salmonella*, among others.

These bacterial colonies form biofilms to protect their residents and keep other bacterial colonies from encroaching on their territory. Whether the biofilm is made of probiotics or conbiotics, they create strong communities the longer they are in place. Biofilms aren't just the bacteria alone; they're also a complex of sugars and protein molecules that create a mucus to bind the bacterial colony together. One common

---

67   Sachin Patel, in conversation with the author, April 20, 2019.

example of a biofilm is the plaque we find on our teeth that creates cavities. The same action is at work among the biofilms in our gut.

The longer the bacterial colony has been in place, the harder it is to break down, which is what makes it so difficult to recover from chronic infections like Lyme's disease. Antibiotics are able to kill the fast-multiplying bacteria, but they don't work against the biofilm.

However, there are ways to break down these biofilms, and the cleansing practices we discuss in the next chapter are effective at breaking down conbiotic communities and helping the body rebuild probiotic communities. One specific method that Dr. Tejero called out was castor oil, which not only breaks down biofilms in the gut, but acts as an anti-inflammatory as well as delivering nutrients to your body.[68]

When the microbiota is thrown off balance, pathogenic bacteria can begin to take over. The microbiota can be disrupted by a variety of factors. Foods that cause inflammation or don't work well for a person's individual system—most commonly processed dairy, modern wheat, alcohol, and lots of refined sugar—can cause an overgrowth of harmful bacteria.

Pesticides from grains and conventionally grown produce can also cause damage to the gut lining. The most common pesticide, glyphosate, is prevalent in most crops, and it not only destroys the gut lining, but it also reduces enzymes in the gut and esophagus that break down our food.[69]

---

68   Marisol Tejero, in conversation with the author, July 15, 2019.

69   Anthony Samsel and Stephanie Seneff, "Glyphosate, Pathways to Modern Diseases II: Celiac Sprue and Gluten Intolerance," *Interdisciplinary Toxicology*, 2013, 6(4): 159-184.

Antibiotics are one of the most potent disruptors of the microbiome: they wipe out all bacteria indiscriminately, permanently altering the microbiome. In July 2018, the *Journal of the American Medical Association* revealed that you are five times more likely to be prescribed unnecessary antibiotics at urgent care compared to family medicine.[70] *At least* 30 percent of the 80 million prescriptions per year of antibiotics "are given without an appropriate indication."

It can take a long time to build up a wide diversity of bacteria in the gut after taking these medications. As the microbiome is rebuilding, it is more vulnerable to imbalance. When pathogenic bacteria take over, the immune system suffers, digestion takes a dive, mood is affected, and disease can result.

LEAKY GUT DEFINED

When the balance of the microbiome is disrupted, it can also result in a condition called *leaky gut*. In a "leaky" gut, the normal gaps in the microvilli that allow nutrients to be absorbed become deteriorated, creating larger holes that allow harmful substances to leak into the bloodstream. As these foreign substances circulate through the body, the immune system goes into overdrive attacking the foreign invaders, and this can result in autoimmune issues and disease. Combine that with "leaky brain," and we have some serious health issues. Evidence suggests that "glyphosate may interfere with the breakdown of complex proteins in the human stomach," according to a 2013 study, "leaving larger fragments of wheat in the human gut that will then trigger

---

70   Katherine E. Fleming-Dutra, et al, "Prevalence of Inappropriate Antibiotic Prescriptions Among US Ambulatory Care Visits, 2010-2011," *Journal of the American Medical Association*, 2016, 315(17): 1864-73.

an autoimmune response, leading to the defects in the lining of the small intestine."[71]

Diet is one of the primary factors that impacts the diversity of the microbiome and the health of the gut. Another major factor is stress, which can have a huge effect on gut health. Stress alone can cause an overgrowth of bad bacteria.[72] High levels of stress for prolonged periods of time can lead to leaky gut and other autoimmune issues. The typical Western diet, which is high in carbohydrates, animal protein, and animal fat, and low in plant fiber, phytochemicals, and fermented foods, also negatively affects the microbiome. It has been linked to a rise in inflammatory-related diseases, including metabolic and intestinal ailments.[73]

The good news? These issues can be remedied by increasing the diversity and richness of the microbiome. Diet is the primary way to rebalance the microbiome, but other lifestyle habits help, too. Because of their relaxing effects, meditation, exercise, fasting, and good sleep can help build good bacteria back up.

When the microbiome is healthy and balanced, we experience positive effects ranging from a strong immune system to better metabolic fitness and mental clarity. "What makes our bodies so beautiful is that fixing them is usually pretty easy. Nature handles complexity," Sachin Patel notes. "Da Vinci said that the greatest sign of sophistication is simplicity.

71   Ibid, Samsel

72   John R. Kelly, et al, "Breaking Down the Barriers: the Gut Microbiome, Intestinal Permeability and Stress-Related Psychiatric Disorders," *Frontiers in Cellular Neuroscience*, 2015, 9: 392.

73   Anica I. Mohammadkhah, et al, "Development of the Gut Microbiome in Children, and Lifetime Implications for Obesity and Cardiometabolic Disease," *Children*, 2018, 5(12): 160.

And what's more sophisticated than the human body? What should be simpler to take care of than the human body?" The key, of course, is to follow the body's wisdom for what it needs in your diet.

CARING FOR YOUR MICROBIOME

Each person's microbiota is individual, and we don't all respond to the same foods the same way. As we discussed before, one person's medicine can be another person's poison. How do you know which foods work for you? One way is to test your microbiota.

GUT CHECK

There is a chart called the Bristol Stool Form Scale, also referred to as the Bristol Stool Chart. It is a diagnostic medical tool, which classifies stool into seven categories. It can be found very easily online, and you can use it to gauge your intestinal health. I won't break that all down here because the visual chart is more powerful for conveying the issue—but go check it out to get insight into your microbiome.

STOOL SAMPLE ANALYSIS

You can also test your microbiome diversity from home with a company called Viome. When you send a stool sample to Viome, they use artificial intelligence to analyze the sample and send you individualized results, including the various strains of bacteria found in your microbiome, specific foods to eat and avoid based on your bacterial profile, and recommended supplements to support your gut. The test can also offer insight into your metabolic fitness, including how you process glucose and the impact your metabolism has on weight control. Viome also compares your results to the anonymous data of others who have taken the test, so you can see on a graph where your microbiome compares in terms of richness and diversity and metabolic fitness.

You can also get stool sample analysis done by a holistic health practitioner, who can give recommendations for your specific dietary and supplementation needs.

INFLAMMATORY BLOOD MARKERS

Blood tests can also be used to understand the health of the gut. An IgG test, which measures your inflammatory markers in response to specific foods, can point you to which foods cause inflammation in your body. For example, when my son got the IgG test, it showed that he had a high inflammatory response to eggs. My wife and I had been trying to understand why he had so many bowel issues—and we'd been feeding him eggs every morning. Once we got rid of the eggs, all of the gut issues started to melt away.

GENETIC TESTS

Genetic tests, such as MaxGen or 23andMe, can also give you insight into which foods are appropriate for your makeup. As a side note, MaxGen was developed by a group of physicians, and the genetic material and data from each test is destroyed after the results are delivered, to ensure privacy. 23andMe, on the other hand, has been known to sell their data to pharmaceutical companies.

Another option is the GI Map Test offered by Diagnostic

Solutions Lab (available at www.diagnosticsolutionslab.com/tests/gi-map). The results of this test can give you insight into the specific bacteria and pathogens that make up your gut, as well as recommendations related to dysbiosis and intestinal health.

URINE TESTS

Information about gut health can also be determined from urine tests. Intestinal yeast and bacteria excrete organic acids that show up in urine. An organic acids test (OAT) can also give information about how the body is metabolizing compounds, and delivers seventy-five markers to give an overall picture of a patient's health. Another urine test, the Dried Urine Test for Comprehensive Hormones (DUTCH), can give insight into the hormone activity in the body.

SPECIFIC FOODS TO PAY ATTENTION TO

While testing can give you clear results, it's also possible to understand what works for you simply by paying attention to what you eat and how you feel afterward, and by looking at your stool. Processed foods, including dairy, meat, and packaged foods, grains, alcohol, and sugars all tend to be common culprits that, for many people, can lead to damaging the microbiome. As you saw in the example with my son, eggs triggered an immune response. Nightshades can also cause problems for others, as they can create a buildup of uric acid, which can result in gout or kidney stones in some people. Nightshades include tomatoes, peppers, potatoes, and eggplant; after consuming these vegetables, pay attention to whether you feel any increased inflammation in your body. Meat and alcohol build up uric acid as well. Developing this awareness begins with paying attention to the sensations that arise in your body after you eat.

TESTING WITH AN ELIMINATION DIET

The best way to determine what effects certain foods are having on you is to do an elimination diet. Eliminate one type of food at a time for about three weeks and observe how you feel.

If you are experiencing health issues, try cutting out the following foods, one at a time:
- Dairy
- Grains (and most importantly, wheat)
- Junk food

These three foods are the biggest irritants and triggers in the diets of most people. Depending on your own makeup, there may be other foods that cause inflammation or negative side effects; you may try eliminating these additional common culprits:
- Alcohol
- Coffee
- Red meat
- Carbonated drinks
- Nightshades
- Eggs
- Legumes (peanuts, beans, etc.)
- Processed foods with additives and dyes

Once you have a baseline for how your body feels without these foods, you can try reintroducing them one at a time. The first time you try including the food, watch carefully for how you feel. Do you have gut irritation or fatigue? Do you have skin issues, rashes, itches, aches, and pains? Remember that food is meant to fuel you; it's meant to raise your energy. If a food you eat instead takes energy away, then you know it is lowering your vibration. One other simple tool is to rate your experience with the food based on three criteria: does it give me energy, take energy, or is it neutral? This simple rating will help you determine which foods work best for you.

You can play with diet in the same way you play with breathwork or movement exercises: the point is not to follow a specific protocol, but to experiment with your own body, listen to how it responds, and see what works. You can begin by eliminating one food from your diet for three weeks or so and reintroducing it to see how you feel. The purpose of the experiment is to get in tune with your body and get feedback through food.

BUILDING BACK A HEALTHY BIOME WITH PROBIOTICS AND PREBIOTICS

Probiotics can help restore the diversity of gut bacteria, but there are limitations to how much they can help. Through a stool sample test with a holistic health practitioner or a service like Viome, you can gain insight into what strains of bacteria may be low, and which ones might need a boost; you can then tailor the specific probiotics you take to support those strains.

Saccharomyces boulardii is a good strain to supplement for most people who are taking a round of antibiotics. Taken orally, you can boost concentrations of *Saccharomyces boulardii* in the gut for a short period of time to assist the gut, though the bacteria will be eliminated within a few days. This strain of bacteria facilitates production of lactic acid and B vitamins, while also reducing the growth of harmful yeasts.[74]

Biome Medic, a particular probiotic supplement, has received third party verification that it reduces levels of glyphosate in the body.[75] I have also taken MegaSporeBiotics, a probiotic that offers a variety of strains to rebuild the microbiome. Another way to support and supplement the balance of healthy bacteria in your microbiome is to include naturally-fermented foods in your diet. Foods like kombucha, sauerkraut, kimchi, apple cider vinegar, raw kefir and yogurt contain beneficial bacteria that can support and restore the diversity of the microbiome.

You can make your own kefir from raw cow or goat milk, or even coconut water. Cow's milk tends to be harder for many people's digestive systems to break down, but when it's fermented as kefir, it becomes much easier to digest, and it feeds the gut with good bacteria.

INCREASING GCMAF

I have used Bravo yogurt in my diet: Bravo yogurt contains many more strains of bacteria than other varieties of yogurt,

---

74 Antonella Gagliardi, et al, "Rebuilding the Gut Microbiota Ecosystem," *International Journal of Environmental Research and Public Health*, 2018, 15(8): 1679.

75 "Groundbreaking Detox Product Shown to Reduce Levels of Glyphosate in the Body," *Sustainable Pulse*, May 30, 2018.

and it stimulates the production of GcMAF. GcMAF is a protein molecule, which is produced naturally in healthy people. It helps regulate and initiate eleven neurological and cellular functions, and it is responsible for activating macrophages. The word *macrophage* is derived from *macro,* meaning "big," and *phage,* meaning "eater." Macrophages "eat" toxins, viruses, tumors, and unhealthy cells. If the immune system becomes depleted or compromised, the body can stop or limit production of GcMAF, which in turn will stop activating the macrophages and therefore allow disease and viruses to proliferate.

Bravo yogurt can be used to help activate GcMAF, as well as provide good bacteria to the gut, and you can make it at home or order it online. Bravo yogurt is great for anyone, but particularly for people dealing with gut issues.

PREBIOTICS

In addition to probiotics to restore the diversity of bacteria strains in the gut, we also need *prebiotics* to feed the good bacteria. We can get the two most important prebiotics, inulin and fiber, through diet. Fresh fruits and vegetables contain a good amount of fiber and inulin to feed gut bacteria, and garlic and artichoke are particularly good sources. Garlic is also anti-parasitic, and it can kill off bad bacteria and yeast. This makes it an especially great food for feeding good bacteria while counteracting pathogens.

Some of the most effective prebiotic foods include:

- Raw garlic
- Raw chicory root

- Raw Jerusalem artichoke
- Dandelion greens
- Raw or cooked onions
- Raw asparagus
- Raw banana

It's recommended to take about five grams of prebiotics per day to support the microbiome, especially if you need to rebuild the microbiome. I like raw onions and garlic, so I frequently mix those ingredients into my cucumber salads, along with apple cider vinegar, which is a fermented probiotic that helps with digestion. I don't feel the need to measure the amounts of these ingredients—with a diet full of fruits and vegetables, I naturally tend to get a good variety of prebiotics and hit the five-gram-per-day mark without effort.

REPAIRING A DAMAGED MICROBIOME

It's possible to repair a damaged gut with these diet recommendations. But for some people whose gut issues are more severe, there is a lot of promising science currently being done on fecal transplants.

A fecal transplant involves taking fecal matter of a person who has a healthy, diverse microbiome and transplanting that into a person who has gut problems, such as Crohn's disease or irritable bowel syndrome. Earlier, we discussed the effect the microbiome has on neurotransmitters and brain health, and studies on fecal transplants are beginning to show the effect this treatment can have on mental functioning. A recent study at Arizona State University tracked children with autism who were given fecal transplants: two years after the transplants, the children reported notable improvements in function.[76]

As one study described, using feces to treat disease is not a recent development:

> As early as 4th century China, suspensions of feces were used to treat food poisoning. Following suggestions from the Bedouins, during the Second World War in Africa, German soldiers adopted the consumption of fresh camel feces as a remedy for bacterial dysentery. In 1958, Ben Eiseman, an American physician, treated four patients affected by pseudomembranous colitis with fecal microbiota transplant (FMT). The first successful treatment of a *Clostridium difficile* infection (CDI) by FMT was documented in 1983.[77]

Microbiologist Lauren Peterson studies the differences in microbiomes between athletes and non-athletes, and she found a distinct difference in balance of gut bacteria among elite athletes like cyclists. Peterson made headlines when she gave herself a fecal transplant from a professional cyclist and saw a noticeable improvement in her ability to train for longer periods of time and at greater intensity.[78] Was it her belief creating the placebo effect, or did it really help? The question remains. Another study showed that athletes with higher levels of cardiorespiratory fitness also had higher

---

76 Dianne Price, "Autism Symptoms Reduced Nearly 50 Percent Two Years After Fecal Transplant," *Arizona State University*, April 9, 2019.

77 Ibid, Gagliardi

78 Marissa Payne, "Move Over, Blood Doping; Cyclists Might Be 'Poop Doping' Soon," *The Washington Post*, June 21, 2017.

levels of diversity in their microbiome.[79] With these early experiments, we're just beginning to see the huge effects that the microbiome can have on one's entire physiology.

Fecal transplants can be done in pill form through companies like OpenBiome. Oral probiotic supplementation only provides a temporary effect. Longer-lasting results can be achieved with fecal microbiota transplants into the colon. There are two or three clinics in the world that do these procedures. In addition to the clinic at Arizona State University, a clinic called Tantamount in the Bahamas provides fecal transplants. It can take multiple treatments per day over a two-week period or more to establish different flora in the microbiome, depending on the issue.

It's important to be cautious about the source of the transplant, as the donor's microbiome will have a huge effect on the recipient's overall health and physiology. In one example, a recipient who was skinny took a fecal transplant from someone who was overweight, and they gained weight after the treatment.

Ozone enemas, which we discussed in chapter three, can also help heal the colon, kill off pathogens, and make room for good bacteria. While there is a lot of promising research beginning to be done in this area, there are still many factors of this kind of treatment that we don't fully understand.

ORTHO BIOTICS AND ESSENTIAL OILS

The prefix *ortho* means "straight," "right," or "correct." Ortho

---

79 Mehrbod Estaki, et al, "Cardiorespiratory Fitness as a Predictor of Intestinal Microbial Diversity and Distinct Metagenomic Functions," *Microbiome*, August 8, 2016.

biotics are essential oils that assist in making the microbiome "right again" by bringing diversity and richness to the bacterial populations in the gut. Ortho biotics target specific strains to prevent the proliferation and accumulation of bacteria and pathogens in the gut. They also help the good bacteria in the gut establish a barrier against pathogens. As opposed to antibiotics, which kill all bacteria indiscriminately (a lose-lose outcome), essential oils can be used to bring bacterial populations into balance (a win-win).

All essential oils are antibiotics. I used a specific essential oil called Flox Detox as one of my first treatments when I began detoxing fluoroquinolones. I also used three different bottles of Doterra essential oils, which I still use to this day. One was called digestZen, which is a blend that is great for anyone with digestion issues; another great digestion blend is called DDR Prime; and the third essential oil is frankincense. I started off using very small amounts of each: I mixed one drop each of digestZEN and frankincense and three drops of DDR Prime with a carrier oil like coconut oil and rubbed it on the bottoms of my feet. The feet have over 200 nerve endings, which help transport the oils to the rest of the body quickly. If you decide to try essential oils for yourself, be sure to get high-quality, 100 percent organic, pure essential oils.

EATING INTUITIVELY

The diet that works for you now may not be the same diet you need over a lifetime. Your body's needs will change over time, and it's important to continually pay attention to what works and what doesn't. The common saying "everything works until it doesn't" applies equally to adaptation and to diet.

In the same way that your body adapts to a workout or a movement exercise, it also adapts to your diet. If you eat the same foods every day, the diet that once felt amazing will lose its effectiveness over time. The body already has the nutrients it needs from those foods, and it may be missing out on other vitamins and minerals. Additionally, eating the same foods consistently can cause the body to create immune responses to those foods over time. The ability to eat the same foods all the time is a modern phenomenon. As hunter-gatherers, humans used to eat whatever they could get their hands on, and the availability of foods changed with the day and the season. Our diet is meant to come from numerous and varied natural sources.

No dietary advice is cut and dry. Rather than following a set of specific guidelines, it's best to eat intuitively. In nature, humans and animals eat with the seasons. Just as you change up the exercises in your workout to build your muscles in different ways, you want to periodically shake up the foods in your diet to get different nutrients. It's best to cycle foods in and out to get a wide diversity in your diet. Remember that during winter, certain trees stop growing, certain animals go into hibernation and your body will do the same with certain seasons. You may not feel like training as intensely during the winter because your body is adapted for reduced activity, whereas as soon as spring hits you may jump into higher workout mode. Similarly, your intuition will guide you to choose different foods at different times depending on the season and your body's needs.

Ask yourself: *Does this food sit well with me? Does it make me feel good? How do I feel throughout the whole process of eating it? Does it bring me happiness during and after eating?*

THE PROBLEM WITH PESTICIDES

As we discussed earlier, pesticides, which are prevalent in conventionally grown crops, can damage the villi in our intestinal lining. These synthetic chemicals can deteriorate the gaps in the intestinal lining and lead to leaky gut. As toxins slip through the gaps, fat-soluble toxins can get stored in the fat, while water-soluble toxins can circulate in the blood, bone, lymph, connective tissue, and joints. Remember, the first step to healing is to eliminate the things that created the issues in the first place; pesticides are one of the main culprits because they are acidic and poisonous to the body.

"THE DIRTY DOZEN"

A habit I would highly recommend considering is staying away from conventional crops that are sprayed with pesticides. A list of the "Dirty Dozen," put together by the Environmental Working Group (EWG), ranks the foods that have the highest pesticide content. They take food samples of various crops and measure the pesticide content, and the foods with the highest concentrations make the "dirty dozen" list. For example, EWG says that roughly 70 percent of the kale samples they collected were tainted by possible cancer-causing chemicals. It's best to avoid the foods on the following list, or buy organic. The list changes every year as foods are continually assessed. You can find updates on the EWS website: https://www.ewg.org.

Aside from following the Dirty Dozen, you can also gauge what foods are likely to contain pesticides based on how exposed they are to the elements. For example, a banana is covered by a peel, so if that crop is sprayed with pesticides, the chemicals are not going to penetrate that fruit as badly as something like celery, which has no layer of protection. The shell of an avocado keeps it protected from pesticides. With berries, on the other hand, the chemicals are directly applied to the part of the fruit that is eaten. Some of these compounds remain even after the fruit is washed. So the food that could potentially be medicine can be neutralized by the poison of the pesticides.

One trick for removing pesticides from produce is to soak the food in either apple cider vinegar or a solution of baking soda and water. Baking soda is alkaline: it kills bacteria, and it's an excellent neutralizer for pesticides and other chemicals. (For example, it can neutralize bee stings and fire ant bites which is a quick hack: as soon as you get bit by any insect, even a mosquito, mix baking soda and white vinegar and apply it to the bite. The faster you put it on, the less reaction you will have.) Mix baking soda and water and splash your produce around in the solution, then rinse the produce.

THE EFFECTS OF GENETICALLY MODIFIED ORGANISMS

Genetically Modified Organisms (GMOs) are developed for numerous reasons, but some are engineered to either resist pesticides, so that the crops can be sprayed liberally with chemicals to control pests, or they are manipulated so that pesticides are grown in the actual food. In the second instance, when a bug goes to bite into the food, the pesticide in that crop causes the bug to die.

If GMOs are designed to do that to bugs, what do you think these compounds do to us? The human gut is able to tolerate these chemicals better than a bug's system can, but we're only able to tolerate these substances for so long. These pesticides will eventually deteriorate the intestinal lining and are linked to leaky gut, as well as cancer.[80] In fact, just this year, a major lawsuit was won against Monsanto (recently acquired by Bayer) due to their pesticides causing cancer. Bayer was ordered to pay more than $2 billion to a couple who said their diagnosis of cancer was given after using the weed killer and pesticide glyphosate.[81] If you continually eat GMOs and expose yourself to pesticides, you're asking for health issues.

Many countries have banned GMO foods because of the health effects and the unknown long-term consequences, but the US hasn't. However, we should soon see labeling to identify which foods are GMO and which ones are not. That we have to ask whether food is organic or not is just another indicator of how far removed from nature we are. We should never have to ask that question in a healthy society where people know the risk of disconnecting from the roots of our past.[82]

ELIMINATING ALCOHOL

I drank heavily in my younger years, but I gave up alcohol at age twenty-two when I realized it did nothing good for me (or for anyone else, as far as I saw). As a coach and trainer, I always suggest removing alcohol as one of the first steps of healing or improving the results of a training program, and I have endless examples of dramatic transformations I've

---

80 Ibid, Samsel

81 Paul Elias, "Jury Orders Monsanto to Pay $2 Billion in Roundup Weed Killer Cancer Case; Appeal Expected," *USA Today*, May 13, 2019.

82 Behrokh Mohajer Maghari and Ali M. Ardekani, "Genetically Modified Foods and Social Concerns," *Avicenna Journal of Medical Biotechnology*, 2011, 3(3): 109-117.

seen people undergo—mentally, emotionally, spiritually, and physically—all from the removal of this one poison and the addition of some honest introspection.

Alcohol is a nervous system depressant, so it slows the brain's impulses as they travel out to the peripheral nervous system. Movement is dramatically affected by alcohol because alcohol can slow down signals to the peripheral nervous system, as well as impair motor control. Alcohol can cause fewer muscle fibers to be recruited, which means fewer results in physical training, in addition to an increase in the chances of injury.

The effects of alcohol last even after alcohol is metabolized. This is why pilots can't drink for twenty-four hours leading up to a flight. In one study, a group of pilots drank enough alcohol between six and nine p.m. to raise their blood alcohol levels (BAC) between 0.10 and 0.12, while another group of pilots consumed a placebo. The next morning, even after they'd slept and their BAC had returned to zero, the pilots that drank had impaired performance in a flight simulator, compared to the placebo group.[83]

Alcohol is also an appetite stimulant, and it spikes blood sugar. Alcohol contributes to leaky gut and creates conditions that allow bad bacteria to thrive in the gut—and those bacteria, in turn, cause us to crave crappy foods to sustain that environment. Because the gut is directly connected to the brain, alcohol can also be a culprit in leaky brain as well. The crazy part is that, not only is alcohol a poison to the body, it also produces a poison as it is being metabolized. Alcohol is not metabolized like most food and drink; it gets absorbed by

---

83 Timothy Roehrs and Thomas Roth, "Sleep, Sleepiness and Alcohol Use," *National Institute on Alcohol Abuse and Alcoholism.*

the gut. Since it is a poison, what is the body's first priority? To get rid of the poison ASAP. That means all the body's other processes, from healing to the fat burning that your body wants and needs to perform, is no longer a priority. The task of metabolizing alcohol adds to the allostatic load of issues the body is already working on.

Alcohol also affects sleep patterns. When alcohol is in the system, we don't go into a deep REM recovery sleep.[84] This prevents our bodies from being able to fully rest and repair. Quality sleep is one of the most important things as it pertains to healing, health, recovery, and even weight loss. As a coach, we ask two primary questions of people who want results: How is your sleep? And how is your water intake? If these two crucial elements are not in order, then good luck healing, burning fat, getting stronger, achieving any number of results; the list can go on and on.

In addition to robbing the body of deep, restorative sleep, one study showed that alcohol consumption increases sleep apnea and decreases oxygen saturation in asymptomatic men—meaning that men who had no symptoms of illness had reduced oxygen levels and an increase in irregular breathing patterns just from consuming alcohol.[85] Alcohol consumption is linked to back pain, a correlation that makes complete sense to me as a back pain relief expert. When alcohol is consumed, specific neurotransmitters do not get released, and this causes more tension, inflammation, and increased blood pressure and stress on the body.

---

84 I. O. Ebrahim, et al, "Alcohol and Sleep I: Effects on Normal Sleep," *Alcoholism: Clinical and Experimental Research*, 2013, 37(4): 539-549.

85 Carole White, et al, "Alcohol Increases Sleep Apnea and Oxygen Desaturation in Asymptomatic Men," *American Journal of Medicine*, 1981, 71(2): 240-245.

These effects are just scratching the surface. In one study, "average" alcohol consumption was found to increase the risk of a long list of chronic diseases: mouth and oropharyngeal cancer; oesophageal cancer; liver cancer; breast cancer; unipolar major depression; epilepsy; alcohol use disorders; hypertensive disease; hemorrhagic stroke; and cirrhosis of the liver.[86]

If you're looking for healing, optimal health, peak performance, mindset, and recovery, cutting out poison (alcohol) is a crucial first step.

THE RITUAL OF EATING

Equally important as the foods we eat is the process our bodies go through to assimilate the nutrients in them. We need a relaxed, calm environment to activate our parasympathetic nervous system in order to digest optimally. The *way* we eat and the rituals we establish around meals are an important component of our overall health.

Think of the difference between your grandma's home cooking and a meal hastily whipped up on the go. Grandma's cooking is amazing because it's made with love, care, and attention—she puts positive energy into creating the meal. When we grab food in a hurry, we often feel anxiety or frustration around what we're eating, and the stress of that experience affects our ability to appreciate as well as absorb and digest the nutrients in that food.

Every thought and feeling we have creates a cascade of chemi-

---

86 Jurgen Rehm, et al, "The Relationship of Average Volume of Alcohol Consumption and Patterns of Drinking to Burden of Disease: An Overview," *Addiction*, August 27, 2003, 98(9).

cals in our brain and in our gut. If we approach a meal feeling angry, irritated, stressed out, or anxious, the energy of those emotions carries into how we digest, assimilate, and process our food. Instead, we want to sit down to each meal feeling relaxed, calm, and grateful. The energy of those emotions helps us digest and reap the full benefits of our food.

Recognize the story and emotions associated with what you are eating. Is there guilt and shame? Are you forcing yourself to eat something that you don't like? Do you say, "I shouldn't be eating this, but..."? All these things affect the cells and the digestion process. This is why prayer over food is so powerful: It is usually an expression of gratitude before beginning a meal. These rituals have a positive effect on our energy as we eat and digest. I suggest to my clients that they take ten slow, deep breaths before each meal to bring them back to the present moment; next, I tell them to share a thought of gratitude for what they are eating. This simple exercise takes one minute and can dramatically alter the mindset and physiology of the body to instantly benefit digestion.

DR. EMOTO AND THE EFFECT OF EMOTIONS ON FOOD

Researcher Dr. Masaru Emoto conducted experiments to understand whether our emotions and words have an effect on the substances around us, including our water and our food. Dr. Emoto put out three glass beakers of rice and then filled them with water. Then, every day for a month he said, "Thank you," to one, and, "You're an idiot," to another. He ignored the third beaker. After a month, the beaker he said, "Thank you," to began to ferment and had a strong pleasant smell. The rice in the beaker to which he'd said, "You're an idiot," turned black. The beaker that was ignored began to rot.

Dr. Emoto ran similar experiments with water: he took samples of polluted water from the Fujiwara dam, froze them, and took pictures of the ice crystals that developed. The crystals of polluted water were ugly and distorted. He took additional samples from the same water source, had people pray over them, and froze that water—and the resulting ice crystals were beautiful, symmetrical snowflakes. Through prayer and intention, he concluded, people could change the structure of the water.

Consider what this might mean for the food and water you take into your body. If you don't have the money or resources to fill your diet with fresh, organic foods, the energy you put into preparing your food with love and joy can have an effect on how your body assimilates that nutrition. In fact, you have the power to make low vibrational food transmute into higher vibration with the thoughts, feelings, and energy you give towards it.

SAVOR THE PROCESS

As soon as you smell food you're about to eat, you've already begun the digestion process. The smell of food stimulates the salivary glands and digestive chemicals in the gut. In fact, the gut can decipher from the smell of food what specific chemicals will be needed to break down the foods we're about to eat, and it tailors that chemical cocktail to each specific meal.[87] The smell of food also brings up specific emotions

---

87 Claus Brandt, et al, "Food Perception Primes Hepatic ER Homeostasis via Melanocortin-Dependent Control of mTOR Activation," *Cell*, November 15, 2018, 175(5): 1321-35.

and thoughts, and we begin to tell ourselves a story about the food we're about to eat and the effect we think it will have on us. As you saw in chapter two, our stories become our beliefs, and they affect our energy and actions in the world. The stories we tell ourselves around our food are as important as the food itself.

There is a saying that a good beginning is half the battle, and this is so true as it pertains to food. Long before the food touches your tongue, your body prepares to ingest it. There are three phases of digestion: the cephalic phase, the gastric phase, and the intestinal phase.

The Cephalic Phase

The cephalic phase starts with the thoughts, sights, and smells of food, which trigger a cascade of events to prepare the body for ingesting and digesting. During the cephalic phase, the vagus nerve that connects the brain to the gut is stimulated, which causes the stomach to secrete digestive enzymes.

I am certified in hypnotherapy, and we use what's called the "lemon test" to determine a person's susceptibility to hypnosis. The test measures how well you can visualize and react to those visualizations, and it's a clear illustration of what happens during the cephalic phase. When doing the lemon test, we have a person picture themselves sitting in a comfortable place in their home. We then have them imagine that they stand up, go into their kitchen, open the fridge, and feel a waft of cold air on their skin. Inside the fridge, we have them picture a bowl of bright yellow lemons, and walk them through the steps of taking a lemon out and slicing into it. At the end of the visualization, we have them imagine taking a big, juicy bite. Most people have visceral reactions to the end of this exercise: they pucker their faces, their eyes water, and they wince and pucker their lips. Those thoughts alone started the digestion process. This is a perfect example of how thoughts and emotions create physical stimulations and give clear indication about how thoughts and feelings manifest our reality.

The Gastric Phase

The next phase is the gastric phase, in which a cascade of chemical and physiological events occurs to activate stomach reflexes and secretory activity. The vagus nerve is stimulated in this phase as well, and if there is emotional distress while you are eating and the fight-or-flight response is still active, the parasympathetic response that allows your body to "rest and digest" is overridden. In this state, food doesn't get broken down and assimilated like it should. The body always gives priority to the built-in survival mechanism of fight and flight. Also, if there is excessive acidity in the stomach, gastric secretion can decline. Food can putrefy and ferment in the gut, which can lead to leaky gut.

Taking into account the widespread use of medications and pesticides; increased intake of meats, alcohol, and processed foods, the reduction in dietary fibers; and the prevalence of emotional stress, can you start to see why so many people today suffer from digestive issues?

The Intestinal Phase

The final phase is the intestinal phase, in which the digestive waste is eliminated. Now, I am no scientist, but my inkling is that if the first two phases don't go well, then this phase will be more challenging. Essentially, in this phase the contents of the stomach begin to empty into the duodenum, which stimulates another cascade of chemicals and physiological processes that allow the body to eliminate stool.

ON EATING SLOWLY

I believe it was the famous holistic wellness coach Paul Chek who said we should drink our food and chew our liquid. He recommends chewing food until it's liquid in the mouth, and when drinking liquids, let them sit in the mouth and "chew" on them. By doing this, you let the tongue, teeth, and tissues in your mouth touch and taste your food, and this helps the stomach prepare more fully for digestion. It also is indicative of conscious eating or eating with the intention of good digestion.

When you eat big chunks of food too quickly, they don't get digested properly, and the nutrients in them aren't fully absorbed. Your stomach will struggle to produce enough enzymes to break down that food effectively. If, on top of that, you're not taking time to rest after each meal, your body doesn't have the time to digest fully. Undigested food that passes from the stomach to the gut can be irritating to the gut lining and can lead to leaky gut.

One big shift I had to make in my own eating habits was to slow down for meals. Growing up, my family ate fast—we would just shove food down our throats. As I started my healing journey with severely damaged intestines and became more connected to true health, healing, and serving my body,

I had to learn to change how I ate dramatically. I could no longer eat quickly; I realized the effect it had on my digestion. I had to sit down, think about my food, chew it fully until it was liquid, and then swallow it.

I'm now helping my son with the same practice. When I see him shovel food in his mouth, I tell him, "Roman, we're going to play a game. I want you to see if you can chew 30 times for every bite." (He often responds to this game by chewing very fast, but at least he's chewing thoroughly.)

The rituals we hold around our meals create the atmosphere in which we accept nutrients and digest. When you create a relaxed experience in which you can hold gratitude for your food, it makes a big impact on your gut health, your energy levels, and how you feel after you eat.

Gratitude is so important. Today we have food that is just readily available, but I want you to think about what it would be like and the appreciation you would have for your food if you had to personally take every step to stalk, kill, butcher, transport, and store the meat of each animal you and your family ate. What if you had to farm, hunt, and harvest every ingredient of the meal that finally ends up on your dinner table? The level of gratitude and appreciation you feel for your food would be dramatically different. Try to connect with that feeling when you eat anything—because it took time and energy for someone to cultivate it or a life was given so yours can live on.

THE HACKS

Accessible Methods

- Look to where your food comes from and try to get as close as possible to the source, so that you can fill your diet with live, energy-rich, and nutrient-dense foods.
- Include fermented foods and prebiotic foods in your diet.
- Use the elimination diet to determine which foods are triggers for you.
- Buy organic whole foods.
- Wash produce that may have been exposed to pesticides with a baking soda solution or apple cider vinegar.
- Create rituals of relaxation and gratitude around mealtimes. Start with ten deep, slow breaths in through the nose, filling up the belly.

Advanced Methods

- Get a test of your inflammatory markers (IgG) to understand what elements of your diet are causing inflammation.
- Take a simple at-home genetic test, such as 23andMe or MaxGen, to understand more about your gut health.
- Use the Viome test to gain insight into the bacteria in your gut and the foods that work best for your microbiome, or get a stool sample tested by a holistic health practitioner.
- Look into fecal transplants to heal a severely imbalanced microbiome.

Things to Consider Avoiding
- Alcohol.
- Eliminate or reduce the amount of pesticides in the foods you eat.
- Angry, anxious, stressed thoughts, and emotions prior to or during eating.

CHAPTER SIX

OUT WITH TOXINS, IN WITH HEALING

In today's society, we're burdened by an abundance of toxins. From car fumes to perfumes to water treatment chemicals and neurotoxic flame retardants in our furniture, our bodies are inundated every day with substances that don't belong in our systems. Everyone, at some point, needs a detox—if you live in modern society, there is no escaping it.

Our digestive systems do the brunt of the work to process these harmful substances out of our bodies. As we discussed in the last chapter, our microbiome helps break down all the foods and substances we ingest so that we can absorb their nutrients and dispose of wastes. The digestive system, liver, and kidneys can get overloaded, and they need periodic cleansing to clear out toxins that build up over time.

In this chapter, we'll look at several different protocols for detoxing the gut—but as I learned through my own healing journey, our digestive health doesn't begin with the gut. We have to begin by looking much farther up the line.

HEALTH BEGINS WITH THE MOUTH

Chinese medicine recognizes that every part of the mouth is connected to other organs and systems of the body. If one part of the mouth is afflicted with an issue, another organ in the body may be suffering, too. In the Chinese system, as in reality, everything is connected.

Mercury is a known neurotoxin, and yet, it's a common component of silver amalgam fillings—which means many of us have this poison in our mouths. Every time a person with amalgam fillings chews food or drinks hot liquid, the mercury off-gasses, and the mercury vapors are absorbed into the body.[88] Amalgam fillings are banned in twenty-eight countries to protect people, especially children and pregnant mothers, against their ill effects.[89]

That's why, when I began working with David Jack at the beginning of my healing journey, one of his first questions was whether I had any amalgam fillings.

The dentist I went to growing up was liberal with fillings. My mom, dad, and sister all have several teeth that were drilled and patched with amalgam fillings, and I had a mouthful of them. When I later realized I might be having health problems associated with the mercury in those fillings, my dad went back to that dentist and asked him about it. The dentist insisted there was no problem with the mercury in his mouth. It wasn't the dentist's fault, of course; he was taught by people who assured him that this was the best way to treat

---

88 Anya Vien, "FDA Has Known for Years: Silver Fillings Cause Kidney, Brain, Urological, Fertility, Neurological and Renal Problems," *Anya Vien* (blog), September 6, 2018.

89 Alireza Panahpour, "28 Countries Ban Mercury 'Silver' Fillings for Children and Pregnant Mothers," *The Systemic Dentist*, February 18, 2018.

teeth. (The holistic dentist I eventually went to, on the other hand, became a holistic dentist because he'd suffered two heart attacks, which he connected to his mercury exposure from amalgam fillings.)

And yet, among all the symptoms I'd experienced during my illness, one notable issue was an acute pain in the back of my head. For two or so years, the pain was consistent and sharp, as though someone was stabbing me in the brainstem with an ice pick. At the time, I didn't know what this pain was from, and I couldn't find relief from it.

When I told David Jack that I had eight amalgam fillings in my teeth, he was astonished. He explained that the mercury in my fillings was one of the factors keeping me sick, and he recommended I get them removed as quickly as possible. I took immediate action, and went to a dentist to have all of my fillings drilled out.

The dentist didn't see a problem with removing the fillings all at once. I was ignorant to the proper way to remove fillings, so it didn't strike me as odd that the dentist didn't use a dental dam or a vacuum to remove the toxic fumes as he removed the mercury fillings. I remember sitting in the chair as they drilled the fillings out of my teeth, and chips of the amalgam material shot into the back of my throat. I have no doubt that I ingested quite a bit of mercury during the procedure.

I would later find out this was not the way to get them removed; I should have gone to an IAOMT-certified holistic dentist. The dentist told me not to worry, that taking them all out at once, even with pieces flying around, was no issue.

But given the amount of mercury in my system at that time, this was a tremendous task, and the detoxification process, as you'll see shortly, came with some serious consequences.

Even so, as soon as the fillings were out, the stabbing pain in my brainstem was dramatically reduced. As soon as I stepped out of the dentist's office, I felt some semblance of relief from this pain that had plagued me for years. It wasn't completely gone, but it had dissipated to a great degree. Looking after the health of my mouth was one of the first major steps to improving the health of my whole body.

HOLISTIC MOUTH CARE

Like David Jack, whenever I am approached by someone who feels ill and can't figure out the problem, or has been diagnosed with Lyme, fibromyalgia, or another autoimmune disease, one of the first questions I ask is whether they have amalgam fillings.

Andy Cutler, a research scientist with a PhD in chemistry from Princeton and former NASA employee, cured his own mercury poisoning and then made his findings available to the world through his books. In addition to creating the Cutler Protocol (detailed later in this chapter), he wrote a book called *Amalgam Illness Diagnosis and Treatment: What You Can Do to Get Better and How Your Doctor Can Help*. On the cover of the book, he attributed almost every serious illness you can think of to mercury toxicity.

On one of the healing retreats I hosted in Costa Rica, I asked the group if anyone had amalgam fillings, and the two who responded with a yes both had chronic autoimmune issues.

One of them had Crohn's disease, which is associated with mercury poisoning. The other participant had Lyme disease. It was clear to me that the overall health of these participants was connected in part to the health of their mouths. Same with root canals; many illnesses are directly linked to root canals.

REMOVING AMALGAM FILLINGS THE RIGHT WAY

If you have amalgam fillings, one of the first steps you'll want to take in your healing journey is to have all fillings removed by a holistic dentist. Specifically, look for a dentist who is certified by the International Academy of Oral Medicine and Toxicology (IAOMT). You can search for a local IAOMT-certified dentist on the academy's website, iaomt.org.

Dentists with this specialized training will know how to take amalgam fillings out safely, and replace them with another non-toxic material, such as porcelain fillings. Amalgam fillings can affect so many of our body's systems that one holistic dentist I go to told me that when women who are having trouble getting pregnant remove their amalgam fillings, their chances of conception go up.

Keeping your mouth healthy and clean is extremely important for the health of the rest of your body and gut. One of the best things you can do for your immune system is to get regular dental cleanings from a holistic dentist.

At home, you can clean your teeth and mouth with all-natural products. While fluoride is generally accepted as a cleaner for teeth, it's actually a cancer-causing toxin. Instead, baking soda and essential oils can be used to neutralize bacteria and toxins and clean the mouth. I use a natural toothpaste that includes a mixture of clay and antibacterial essential oils like clove, oregano and peppermint.

In the last chapter, we discussed the importance of filling your diet with fruits and vegetables, which help maintain a healthy gut. These same foods promote health in the mouth, too. Raw fruits and vegetables contain fiber that scrubs your teeth when you take a bite. Some nutrients are absorbed directly into the gums, tongue, and tissues of the mouth. The mouth is where digestion begins, and by giving proper care and attention to the mouth, we can impact the health of the whole body.

A TEETH, MOUTH, AND THROAT CLEANING HACK

This hack to cleanse the mouth comes with additional benefits: it can pull up mucus from the chest as well as reduce or even eliminate a sore throat.

Put a teaspoon of bentonite clay in two to three ounces of water and set aside.

Oil pull with one teaspoon coconut oil or sesame oil by pulling and pushing the oil through your teeth around in your mouth for ten to fifteen minutes. Once you have done the oil pulling, make sure to spit the oil in the toilet or outside, because it is filled with rancid bacteria.

Next, take a half ounce to an ounce of the clay water in your mouth. Gargle and swish it around for two to three minutes, and spit it out in the toilet or outside. Repeat with the remaining clay, a half ounce to an ounce at a time for three to five rounds. Never swallow the oil or clay after pulling. Bentonite clay is negatively ionized, and toxins have a positive charge, so the clay pulls all the bacteria, mucus and toxins from the mouth (as well as bringing it up from the throat and chest).

In another variation, you can do an oil pull with castor oil, which only needs to be swished in the mouth for roughly one minute to clean the mouth and teeth.

SYSTEM OVERLOAD

"We are living in a toxic world, the world is sick, the world has cancer, the soil is sick, the air is contaminated, all we can do is keep our bodies clean and our self-healing mechanisms strong. No disease can exist in a clean body."

— DR. EDWARD F. GROUP[90]

Our bodies are constantly helping us heal by removing the toxins, chemicals, and heavy metals to which we're exposed.

In addition to clearing these waste products from our systems, our bodies are also constantly at work fighting pathogens, including bad bacteria and parasites. Often, these pathogens are synergistic with toxins: for example, Lyme bacteria may feed off heavy metals and synergize with them to create more health issues. Toxins build up in the tissues of our bodies, and

---

90 Ty Bollinger, *The Truth about Cancer* (docuseries), TTAC Publishing, 2015.

in turn they create inflammatory environments for pathogens to grow.

When toxins aren't eliminated properly, they can cause disease in the tissues where they've built up. Neurological issues, chronic fatigue, joint aches and pains, and autoimmune issues can all be connected to toxins that have accumulated in the body.

There are four primary ways our bodies eliminate toxins— our "exhaust pipes." One is through our skin: wastes are expelled through our pores as we sweat. A second path is through our kidneys, which filter out wastes that we then eliminate in our urine. We also eliminate waste through stool, as our digestive system clears out these substances. The final path is through our airways; some substances, such as alcohol, can get expelled through our breath— which is why the Breathalyzer is used to measure BAC, and why some people choose to use breathwork as a tool to cure hangovers.

In any detoxification process, we first have to get the body to release toxins from the tissues and move them into the bloodstream to be processed and eliminated through one of these four paths. This process has to be done carefully, so that the body can properly eliminate the excess toxins circulating in the blood; otherwise, those toxins can be reabsorbed into the tissues and cause more severe issues.

Unfortunately, this is a lesson I learned firsthand by detoxing too fast for my ill state of health. The sicker you are, the more slowly and carefully you may need to detox. Working with an expert is recommended.

USING FASTING AND CLEANSES TO SUPPORT THE BODY

What is your age on a cellular level?

The way to measure this is to test the length of your *telomeres*, sections of DNA on the ends of your chromosomes. There is a massive amount of evidence and science showing that the length of your telomeres is linked to age-related disease. The longer your telomeres, the longer your life. Factors that impact your telomere length include your environment, lifestyle, genetics, and many of the things we are discussing in this book.

When you are born, the length of your telomeres are typically at their longest. As we age and our cells divide, they lose a little DNA in each split, until they gradually deteriorate. This process is accelerated as we're exposed to more toxins in our environment. I interviewed Dr. Daniel Pompa, and he is a huge promoter of fasting, and he turned me on to the company Teloyears, which allows you to test the length of your telomeres.[91] Fasting is one of the key tools for extending the life of your telomeres.

THE BENEFITS OF FASTING

Every religion has fasting traditions, and no wonder: fasting is a spiritual experience with endless health benefits.

If there is one thing that we know for a fact that extends people's lives, it is consuming low calories. The process of digestion consumes a lot of energy. When we fast, there are

---

91   Daniel Pompa, in conversation with the author, September 13, 2019.

several powerful things that happen. First is the process of *autophagy*, which means "self-eating." Autophagy is your body's way of eating up damaged cells and replacing them with new ones. Engaging in autophagy through fasting plays a huge roll in reducing inflammation and can be a therapeutic strategy for rebooting the entire immune system. Fasting triggers the release of stem cells and can initiate the release of white blood cells which are the "front line" of the army of your immune system.[92] These cells go to battle against bad bacteria, viruses, and other pathogens.

If you have digestive issues, a study done by MIT biologists shows that fasting for twenty-four hours can regain age-related loss of stem cell function. As we age, intestinal stem cells lose the ability to regenerate as quickly as they did when we were younger. This decline in stem cell production can make it tougher to recover from gut trauma, infection, and irritation. Researchers found, however, that twenty-four-hour fasting created as large a benefit for older mice as it did for younger ones.

There are several types of fasting, and in this section we'll focus on only a few: intermittent fasting, juice fasting, and water fasting. These different types of fasting vary in intensity, from intermittent fasting, which can be done every day, to water fasting, which could be done two or so times a year. You want to train how you fast in the same way you would train in a physical program: start off small, and progressively take on more challenges, because the body needs adaptation and energy to fast.

---

92 Suzanne Wu, "Fasting Triggers Stem Cell Regeneration of Damaged, Old Immune System," *USC News*, June 5, 2014.

INTERMITTENT FASTING

Start with intermittent fasting. Intermittent fasting is where you eat only in a six- to eight-hour window. For example, you could eat meals in the hours from eleven a.m. to seven p.m., and fast during the hours outside of that time. You can start with two days a week and build up to more days per week as your body adapts. You can work out while in an intermittent fasted state to help maximize fat burning and cellular function, and increase your levels of human growth hormone (HGH), which is a beneficial anti-aging hormone.[93]

JUICE FASTING

The next progression in fasting is to try a juice fast (also called a smoothie fast), where you only consume fresh vegetable and fruit juice or smoothies and water. The length of time you choose to fast depends on how familiar you are with these processes and how your body responds. Start with three to five days, which studies show is the length of time where stem cells are released and the immune system resets itself. Juice fasting is similar to a reduced-calorie diet (also called mimic fasting), where the daily calorie intake is low enough to create the benefits of fasting.

WATER FASTING

Water fasting is where you only have water. Use your intuition to know when your body is ready for a water fast. When it's calling to you, and when it's in your attention—you hear people mention it, you read about it, and you feel it's something your body needs—you can try a three- to five-day fast a

---

93 Rudy Mawer, "11 Ways to Boost Human Growth Hormone (HGH) Naturally," *Healthline*, September 23, 2019.

couple of times a year. After water fasting, cleansing is recommended to use things like binders, castor oil, and magnesium sulfate to clear out the toxins that come up.

You never want to train and work out when doing something like a water fast for extended periods of time. Intermittent fasting is fine because you're still eating daily, but training during a water fast can interrupt the other processes your body is going through. Training requires your body to focus on repairing muscles, and if you don't have the proteins you need for that repair, it's just another stressor added to the system on top of the fasting. Some people still take digested amino acids to maintain their muscles while fasting. Fasting is a time to rest, recover, and allow the body to do what it needs to do.

THE ROLE OF PARASITES IN DIS-EASE

As the name suggests, anaerobic pathogens can survive in the body without the presence of oxygen. Cancer cells also grow in hypoxic environments where there is a lack of oxygen,[94] which is why hyper-oxygenating the body with breathing techniques is so powerful.

Parasites thrive off of processed foods, heavy metals, and sugars, and they eat first: when you intake food, parasites that live in your gut eat what they need, and you get the leftovers. This can lead to a variety of symptoms for the human host: fatigue, brain fog, dizziness, bloating, nutrient deficiencies, and irritability, among others.

---

94 Devic Slobodan, "Warburg Effect – A Consequence or the Cause of Carcinogenesis?" *Journal of Cancer*, April 26, 2016, 7(7): 817-822.

Parasites and an imbalance of bad bacteria in the gut often go hand in hand. As we saw in the last chapter, the bacteria in your gut are responsible for crucial neurotransmitters to the brain that control your emotions and cravings. Pathogens, then, will cause you to crave the sugar and processed foods they thrive on. An employee of mine had always had an intense sugar craving, so I recommended she do the Hulda Clark parasite cleanse (detailed later in this chapter), and her hunger cravings were dramatically reduced. After her first cleanse, her cravings went down, so she did a second cleanse to further reduce her cravings.

In addition to poor diet, we also get parasites from environmental factors, such as living with pets or kids, and not regularly washing our hands. These parasites can affect a variety of tissues in the body, from tapeworms and hookworms that live in the gut, to liver flukes, to ascaris that can cause asthma.

Because parasites are present in so many areas of the body, they can create a wide variety of symptoms. Gut problems such as unexplained constipation, diarrhea, and persistent gas can be signs of parasites in the gut. Nutrition problems, such as anemia, can be a sign that parasites are getting nutrients before you do. Skin issues can also arise from parasite infection: unexplained rashes, eczema, hives, itching, and even muscle and joint pain can be connected to these pathogens.[95]

A comprehensive stool test or blood test from a holistic doctor can help you understand whether your body is fight-

---

95 P. Zaccone, et al, "Parasitic Worms and Inflammatory Diseases," *Parasite Immunology,* October 2006, 28(10): 515-523.

ing parasites. Specific blood tests can also help you determine whether your immune system has created antibodies for particular pathogens. Endoscopies and colonoscopies can also be used to check for parasites, but these are invasive medical interventions that have potential complications. For example, after getting an endoscopy, I developed ulcers in my throat, which the gastroenterologist brushed off, saying, "It happens sometimes." I've also known people who have almost died from intestinal perforations they got from colonoscopies. Other complications include cardiopulmonary complications, and hemorrhaging.[96]

When you're experiencing health issues, a natural parasite cleanse can be a good place to start to help support your body in healing and generally has no drawback and only benefits. Before beginning any fasting and cleansing protocol, it's important to prepare your body properly and give it the nutrients it needs to process the toxins that are released during a cleanse.

CLEANSING BASICS

Like all of the hacks in this book, the cleanses detailed in this chapter are not one-size-fits-all. Each individual has specific considerations and conditions to take into account before doing a cleanse, and above all, it's important to pay attention to how your body responds as you try different treatments. The cleanses I'll discuss here are basic protocols I found in my research that support healthy organ function and help to clear mucus, acid, and parasites from the body.

---

96 ASGE Standards of Practice Committee, "Complications of Colonoscopy," *Gastrointestinal Endoscopy*, October 2011, 74(4): 745-752.

The following is a list of common cleansing agents and simple practices you can use to cleanse your body of parasites. If you're considering a heftier detoxification protocol like a heavy metal detox, it's important to work with an experienced professional who can look at your unique genetic factors, diet, and gut function, and create a protocol that's specific to your current state of health.

Magnesium Sulfate

Magnesium sulfate, or Epsom salt, can be used internally as a liver and gallbladder flush. Many people mix Epsom salt with water and take it as a cleansing agent after a fast. Dr. Hulda Clark, who pioneered the use of many cleanses, describes proper preparation and dosage of magnesium sulfate on her website; there are specific considerations for people with gut issues and constipation. Some people can be sensitive to ingesting Epsom salt, so it's important to test with small amounts and see how your body feels.

Castor Oil

Castor oil has been used for thousands of years for a multitude of benefits. It is a foundational tool to get your body back in balance. Castor oil helps you relax and destress; assists with better digestion, elimination, and reducing inflammation; provides nutrients including glutathione, a master antioxidant, and omega 6 and 9; increases nitric oxide, breaks down biofilms, and resets your microbial activity.

Castor oil can be taken internally to cleanse the intestines and kill parasites, and it can also be used topically to clear mucus in the form of a "castor pack." You can get wool sheets specifically made for this purpose. Pour a little castor oil on the sheet, put it on your belly, and wrap it with cling wrap to keep it in place. You can sleep with a castor pack every night for a week or two to help process out mucus and toxins after a fast. Castor packs are especially useful for children, for whom taking castor oil internally might be too harsh. It's important to use organic hexane free cold press castor oil, preferably in a glass bottle.

Naturopath Dr. Marisol Tejero, who is nicknamed the "Queen of Thrones" for her work on gut issues, is an expert on castor oil; she and I agree that castor oil packs are the best tools to start with when using castor oil for healing.[97] Dr. Marisol points out that castor oil is especially effective in breaking up biofilm in the gut—more effective than any pharmaceutical drug or chemical biofilm breakdown method.

Castor oil packs reset the microbiome and rebalance the ratios of good and bad bacteria in the gut. When you put on a castor pack, you stimulate your nervous system to relax and release dopamine and oxytocin, an effect Dr. Marisol compares to an "escape button on a computer." Even better, you can get these effects from castor packs placed on the skin, without having to go through the digestive system.

Turpentine (100 Percent Pure Pine Gum Spirits)

I learned about the healing properties of turpentine from Dr. Jennifer Daniels, creator of the turpentine candida cleanse, who would continually ask her patients about the healing remedies their parents and grandparents used. Time and

---

97   Marisol Tejero, in conversation with the author, July 17, 2019.

time again, patients told her that the oldest remedies in their families were to use turpentine, and the relatives who used this folk remedy lived long lives and maintained mental sharpness. Turpentine was a traditional slave remedy, administered by putting a teaspoon of turpentine over three cubes of sugar and then eating it. The sugar in the mixture attracts the parasites and bugs, while the turpentine neutralizes them. In Merck's 1899 pharmaceutical manual, turpentine was mentioned 114 times for its health benefits and as a treatment for numerous diseases.[98]

Natural turpentine is produced by pine trees to protect them from fungus, bacteria, and parasites, and when it's distilled in its pure form, it has the same benefits for us: it's a powerful antifungal and antibacterial—a plant medicine that works with our bodies to restore balance, and which also has terpenes that reduce inflammation and pain.

Turpentine can also be used topically. You want to make sure to purchase pure, 100 percent pine gum spirits. I have used Diamond G Products.

BINDERS

In addition to a cleansing agent, it can be helpful to take a *binder* to support your cleanse. Several different substances, such as activated charcoal, bentonite clay, microsilica, clinoptilolite, or Zeolite, to name just a few, act as binders to toxins in the body, and they absorb toxins so that they can be eliminated. Toxins tend to have a positive ionic charge, and binders have a negative charge, so binders stick to toxins and allow

98 *Merck's Manual of the Materia Medica*, New York: Merck & Co., 1899.

them to be passed through the body with the stool. You can find a list of common binders in the appendix.

It is important to note that since binders are so good at binding toxins, the products themselves can many times be contaminated. I would suggest researching the best products that are tested for contamination. Here are some common binders:

- **Bentonite clay** binds bacteria and toxins and can be particularly useful with poison ivy. It can be used as a mouthwash or taken internally to pull bacteria and toxins out of the gut.
- **Microsilica** is particularly effective for heavy metals like aluminum, and it can be taken internally. Fiji and Volvic brand water both contain natural silica, which is proven to carry aluminum out of the brain through the urine.
- **Chlorella** is a heavy metal binder, and it's also a great source of vitamins, minerals, and amino acids. Take care when using it as a binder, because it can mobilize toxins without fully removing them. That said, my kids take chlorella tablets daily, and my wife took them throughout her pregnancies.
- **Activated charcoal** is used by toxicologists to absorb poisons that have been ingested; it's also helpful in binding molds and other toxins. You can take activated charcoal daily, mixed with water or in capsule form.
- **Modified citrus pectin** has anti-tumor properties, in addition to being great for prostate health. You can mix modified citrus pectin with water and take it internally. One brand I recommend is Econugenics Pectasol C.
- **Enterosgel** is a good mold binder and can be taken orally, mixed with water.

- **Clinoptilolite zeolite** binds heavy metals, viruses, fungal toxins, radioactive materials, fluoride, and some pathogenic bacteria, including *Escherichia coli, Bacillus subtilis, Staphylococcus aureus, Salmonella, Streptococcus mutans, Streptococcus mitis,* and *Pseudomonas aeruginosa.* Recommended brands include Advanced TRS Nano Zeolite, and Cytodetox.
- **Diatomaceous earth** is a natural parasite killer, insecticide, and binder for mycotoxins and other heavy metals. It can be tough on the digestive system, so start with small amounts.

CLEANSING PROTOCOLS FOR FURTHER READING

Irene Grosjean's protocol begins by juicing fresh vegetables and blending fruits for two weeks. This builds up nutrients in the body to charge up the "batteries" and store energy to promote healing and be able to fast and cleanse. Several other healers have developed different methods for cleansing, and the following is a list of some of the most powerful ones I've tried. You can easily find more information on each of these healers and their specific protocols through a simple online search.

HULDA CLARK'S CLEANSES

In her book *The Cure for All Diseases,*[99] Dr. Hulda Clark wrote that all diseases, from high blood pressure to seizures to chronic fatigue syndrome to multiple sclerosis,

---

99 Hulda Clark, *The Cure for All Diseases,* New Century Press, 1995.

resulted from problems at the cellular level, including the activity of parasites. She developed simple, low-cost herbal protocols to kill parasites, which you can readily find by reading her book or researching her work. She developed a series of cleanses to target specific parts of the body: her work lays out directions for a parasite cleanse, a digestive cleanse, a candida cleanse, a kidney cleanse, a liver and gallbladder cleanse, and lastly, a heavy metal cleanse.

Dr. Clark also recognized that cells operate on electricity, and she built a specific device called the Zapper, which she used to target the frequencies of specific parasites. She developed the Zapper in the early days before PEMF therapy was used to treat chronic illnesses, and throughout her career, she helped people heal from serious illnesses by focusing on removing parasites and using a frequency generator like the Zapper. Since then, others have built off her work and created much more sophisticated and impactful devices.

GERSON THERAPY

Developed by German doctor Max Gerson, who treated cancer patients with this protocol, the Gerson Therapy involves juicing whole foods, coffee enemas, dental health, castor oil packs, and bentonite clay. Coffee enemas are an excellent liver cleanse, and help the liver release glutathione, a master antioxidant that stimulates healing. Gerson Therapy also includes supplementation, an important facet we'll cover later in this chapter.

THE CUTLER PROTOCOL

Andrew Cutler created this detox protocol for mercury and heavy metal toxicity. The Cutler protocol begins by building up the body with fruits, vegetables, and the "core four" vitamins and minerals: vitamin C, vitamin E, zinc, and magnesium. Taking specific amounts of the core four for two weeks builds up the immune system and helps prepare the body for eliminating toxins.

After the buildup period, Cutler recommends taking small amounts of alpha-lipoic acid, which is a precursor to glutathione, the master antioxidant. Alpha-lipoic acid helps process toxins out of the body, specifically mercury. The Cutler Protocol can be difficult to follow, as the timing of dosages is very specific, and interspersed with periods of rest. It's important to work with a practitioner who can take your unique health conditions and genetic factors into account to gauge whether this is a suitable protocol for you.

SUPPLEMENTATION TO SUPPORT YOUR SYSTEM DURING DETOX

The body naturally cleans out and eliminates toxins, and each of the protocols in this chapter is designed to support the body in doing its work. Particular nutrients can help open the pathways in our epigenetics that turn on the body's cleansing processes. As was noted in the Gerson and Cutler protocols, the liver produces glutathione that detoxifies harmful substances in the body, and certain nutrients, such as vitamin C and vitamin E, help stimulate glutathione production. Similarly, one of my favorite supplement brands, Dr.

Carolyn Dean's B-Complex vitamin, ReAline, is formulated specifically to help the liver produce glutathione. ReAline assists the body in opening up detoxification pathways naturally, and it's less demanding on the body than other more intense cleanses or purges.

VITAMIN C

Vitamin C is a powerful immune system booster and detoxifier. Humans can only get it through diet, whereas most other mammals produce vitamin C on their own.[100] Fruits and vegetables provide the most bioavailable form of vitamin C (which is another reason why juicing and blending is great), but it can also be supplemented with a high-quality sodium ascorbate or even IV vitamin C, which has produced miracles in healing.

It is important to find high-quality vitamin C, because many supplements are made from black mold or from GMO corn. One great high-quality option is the lypo-spheric vitamin C supplements from LivOn Labs. When you're feeling sick, you can take high doses of vitamin C—a gram packet per hour—and it will rapidly help you feel better. Dr. Frederick R. Klenner, who specialized in orthomolecular medicine, pioneered the use of high-dose intravenous vitamin C. He was inspired by Linus Pauling, another vitamin C researcher, to use vitamin C to neutralize toxins, viruses, and histamines, as well as assist with tissue repair. Klenner estimated that most of the population was walking around with subclinical scurvy, and he believed that natural remedies were safer and more effective than drugs. He used high doses of vitamin C

---

100 Cell Press, "How Humans Make Up for an 'Inborn' Vitamin C Deficiency," *Science Daily*, March 21, 2008.

to treat and heal patients who had been diagnosed with polio, and recommended that anyone who is ill should get large doses of vitamin C while the physician ponders the diagnosis.

MAGNESIUM

Magnesium comes in many forms: citronate, threonate, glyconate, and chloride. Most forms are not highly absorbable. Of the four types, magnesium chloride is the most absorbable form. Magnesium helps with many processes in the body, including the metabolism of proteins, fats, and carbs. Dr. Carolyn Dean has a high-quality supplement of magnesium chloride that I recommend to clients at our training facility. They rave about how much better they feel after taking magnesium chloride: their sleep improves, along with digestion and mental clarity. Dr. Dean studied magnesium for over thirty-five years and wrote a book on it called *The Magnesium Miracle.*[101]

Dr. Carol Dean's ReMag or ReMyte is a magnesium supplement that contains additional core minerals that many people can benefit from. I also recommend Magnesium L-Threonate by LivOn Labs, which studies have proven helps with cognitive function and may improve synapse and neuron function in the brain. Swimming in the ocean is also a great natural way to improve magnesium levels.

ALOE VERA

This superfood is packed with a long list of nutrients:

---

101 Carolyn Dean, *The Magnesium Miracle*, Ballantine Books, 2006.

- Twenty of the twenty-two essential amino acids.
- Folic acid, choline, and vitamins A, C, E, B1, B2, B3 (niacin), B6, B12 (which is necessary for red blood cell production).
- Core minerals including zinc, selenium, calcium, magnesium, chromium, sodium, iron, potassium, copper, and manganese.
- Digestive enzymes, like amylase and lipase, which help break down fat and sugar molecules.
- Brandykinase and salicylic acid, which help reduce inflammation.

All of these elements together make aloe vera a potent food for regulating blood sugar, staving off metabolic disease, and assisting in the detox process. Aloe vera has antibacterial, antiviral, and antifungal properties, making it excellent for exercise recovery and gut healing.

You can take aloe vera internally or topically in a variety of ways. You can eat organic aloe vera by blending it in shakes or in water for gut healing and cleansing. As many people know, aloe vera can be used for sunburns as a rapid healer and cooling agent. You can also rub aloe vera on sore joints to promote recovery, and it can be applied topically for ulcers, Crohn's disease, IBS, colitis, and leaky gut. Cut a 3 x 3" piece of aloe, make little incisions in it, place it on your gut, and wrap cling wrap around it to keep it in place for a few hours.

BLACK SEED OIL

Black seed oil gives the immune system a boost by raising levels of glutathione, the liver's master antioxidant. Black seed oil is such a powerful assist for the immune system that it's been noted to help with everything from autoimmune issues and gastrointestinal problems to cognition, respiratory issues, and metabolic processes. Some scientists have called black seed oil one of the most powerful compounds ever discovered. I am part of a Facebook group called "Black Seed Oil Testimonials," on which you can see incredible feedback on the benefits of this supplement. A high-quality brand is Madre Nature Organic Cold Press Cumin Seed Oil.

NANO AND LIPOSOMAL SUPPLEMENTS

With the improvement of supplement technology, companies are making nano and liposomal forms of supplements, which improves absorption and bioavailability. With these forms, you simply hold the liquid under your tongue as it dissolves.

Nanoceutical Solutions has great products for:

- Nano turmeric (for inflammation).
- Nano glutathione (the body's master antioxidant to detox).
- Nano B12 (vital for building red blood cells, brain support and allergy support).
- Nano vitamin D (for, bone health and immune support).

SUPPORTING ELIMINATION WITH COLONICS AND ENEMAS

When we're detoxing, additional wastes get dumped into the intestinal tract. For some people, this extra load can get caught or trapped in the intestines, and it can be useful to do colonics or enemas while detoxing to help keep things moving. Colonics go all the way through the colon to clean it out, while enemas act only on the lower end of the colon. Both processes can help cleanse the body tremendously.

For a colonic, you'll need to find a local clinic. Someone I know gives colonics for a living, and she has told me that many people feel such dramatic relief and sense of relaxation after the process that they hug her and thank her.

Enemas can be done at home, and there are a variety of resources to consult on how to do it, including Hulda Clark's protocol and the Gerson Therapy. If you do an enema at home, it's important to use only distilled water, and boil the enema bag and equipment to sterilize it after use. You can do an enema with a liter of distilled water, and you can also add ingredients to support your system, such as drops of Lugol's iodine to help flush out parasites; coffee to help the liver; digestive enzymes; or probiotics to give your microbiome a boost.

It's important, as always, to monitor how your body feels throughout all these processes, so that you're not taking on too much at once. You want to make sure your body is able to fully process and eliminate all of the toxins that come up. If you feel terrible throughout the process, you won't want to repeat it—instead, you want the process of bringing your body back to nature to be a sustainable one.

THE HACKS

Accessible Methods
- Clean your mouth regularly with natural, non-fluoride toothpaste, and oil pulling, and bentonite clay.

- Try intermittent fasting and juice fasting.
- Use cleansers and binders to clear parasites and bad bacteria from your system.
- Support your detox with supplements (flip to the appendix for a list of supplements).
- Enemas.

Advanced Methods
- Get amalgam fillings removed by an IAOMT-certified holistic dentist.
- Colonics.
- Use a hyperbaric oxygen chamber while fasting, juicing, and cleansing.

Combining the Hacks
- While doing a juicing, fasting, and detox program, you can also do breathwork daily to help oxygenate your body and stimulate the circulatory system and lymphatic system to process and move wastes through your system. Breathwork and hyperbaric oxygen chamber sessions are even more effective while fasting because your body doesn't have to focus on digestion; it can focus instead on what it needs to heal.
- Do breathwork or hyperbaric oxygen chamber sessions while detoxing to speed up the process of expelling toxins.

Things to Consider Avoiding
- Don't jump into intensive detox practices, like a heavy metal detox, without the guidance of an experienced practitioner.

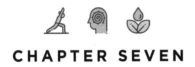

CHAPTER SEVEN

NATURE'S NURTURE

In the midst of my healing journey, when I was still dealing with illness, still overworking myself, and at a loss for what to do, my sister sent me a link to photos of a treehouse community in Costa Rica.

The community looks like an Ewok village. It's up in the mountains, and the elevated houses have hanging bridges and zip lines to connect the community. Dappled sunlight filters through the trees, and there are butterflies all around. It's a magical, almost fairytale world, and a stark contrast to what I was used to in the concrete jungle of New York City where I lived for the latter third of my life before moving to South Carolina.

My soul was yearning for the jungle and was calling me to Central or South America. As soon as I saw a video about the place, I knew I needed to go there, so I booked a flight.

I rented a treehouse, and I felt instantly connected to the jungle and the trees around me. During my childhood, I'd spent hours playing outdoors in the woods. It was part of who I was—and it is part of who everyone is. We are nature.

We are meant to connect with nature as much as possible. It brings us joy, peace, and happiness, and the more we are in that state, the faster we heal and recharge our batteries.

Being in Costa Rica had an instant positive effect on my health. The first benefit I saw was an improvement in my sleep. Before I'd gotten sick, I'd been a deep sleeper. As I got sick, however, I found myself waking up with anxiety at all hours of the night, and then I'd be so exhausted I would pass out in the middle of the day. I was a mess. In Costa Rica, I slept deeper than I had in years. When I woke up, I felt rejuvenated.

While I was there, I looked around at properties to buy, but my dream to own one seemed unrealistic. However, a property owner heard I was looking and decided to cut his price in half to entice a sale, because he owned two lots and wanted to buy a new home in the States. It was the biggest lot in the community, bordered by a big river on one side and a stream on another. I felt so amazing in this environment, and this property becoming available was serendipitous. I felt I had been divinely inspired to come here, like this was where God wanted me to be.

I bought the property.

At the time, I had no idea how I was going to build on the property, or if I would have the money for it. I took a leap of faith. As my business continued to grow and expand, I had more and more resources to return to Costa Rica and build my own tree house.

I built it for three reasons: I wanted my own healing getaway, a place to completely disconnect. I also built it to run fitness transformational retreats, so that I could teach people breathwork and other techniques to heal naturally—some of the transformational techniques I've laid out in this book. And the final reason I built the treehouse was because it could be entirely self-sustaining. The property is completely off the grid. All organic food is grown on site, with a beautiful garden and fruit trees all around. There are fifteen natural springs pumping water; it's like the garden of Eden. If the world collapsed, this property would still be a place of healing and refuge with all of life's necessities.

A DAILY DOSE OF NATURE

As I began bringing clients to Costa Rica, it quickly became clear that I wasn't the only one who craved time in nature and felt healing benefits from it. As people came to visit the treehouse, I saw them arrive feeling fatigued, burned out, stressed, and in need of a lot of healing and connection with self and others. In just a day or two, I saw the same stressed-out, disconnected people open up. Recently, a whole group was brought back to a state of childlike innocence: they were uninhibited, free of judgment, and filled with love, joy, and peace. We were all playing in this garden together like children exploring a new world for the first time. This is exactly the effect I like to see by hosting retreats in nature; I want to see people reconnecting with who they truly are, and to return to a pure state of joy and bliss.

I found nature exposure to be hugely beneficial for healing in my personal experience, and I was interested to find studies done on the effects of nature on the body. I quickly realized that for a few reasons, the specific effects can be hard to measure scientifically. The first challenge is that researchers had to define what they meant by nature. What part of nature would they look at in each study? What people and cultures are interacting with it, and how are they affected? Among these questions, there are a multitude of factors that go into the interaction between people and our environment. Still, studies have shown that spending time in parks and natural spaces in urban environments promotes better health overall.[102]

Another recent study showed that spending twenty minutes a day outdoors dramatically reduces cortisol levels.[103] Cortisol sustains the stress response, and it is necessary and important for specific functions, but modern life and modern society have created conditions that bombard us with constant high levels of stress. When cortisol levels are elevated and sustained, problems can occur.

There are many beneficial physiological effects that occur when humans interact with plants, animals, and wilderness. Studies on gardening have shown that it lowers blood pressure, for example.[104] Multiple studies have shown natural environments to help restore brain function, leading to better concentration, productivity, and a more positive outlook on life.[105]

---

102 Cecily Maller, et al, "Healthy Nature Healthy People: 'Contact Nature' as an Upstream Health Promotion Intervention for Populations," *Health Promotion International*, December 22, 2015, 21(1): 45-54.

103 "Just 20 Minutes of Contact with Nature Will Lower Stress Hormone Levels, Reveals New Study," *Science Daily*, April 4, 2019.

104 Richard Thompson, "Gardening for Health: A Regular Dose of Gardening," *Clinical Medicine*, June 2018, 18(3): 201-205.

105 Alanna Ketler, "Doctors Explain How Hiking Can Actually Change Our Brains," *Collective Evolution*, April 8, 2016.

Additionally, studies have shown that nature-based therapy can often give relief and results to patients who had not responded to other forms of treatment.[106] It was easy to see the positive effect of nature on my children: when they were babies, if they got injured or upset, I would instantly pick them up and take them for a walk in the woods. They would quickly stop crying and become more relaxed. Connecting with the earth and natural environments fosters recovery and restoration. I now make a daily practice out of grounding with the earth. Every day I try to go outside, lay on the grass, and get a little sun. Each time I do this simple practice, I instantly feel more relaxed, revitalized, and restored.

TAKE A NATURE PILL

You can run your own simple experiments on the healing effects of nature: compare what it feels like to do a meditation in a room of your house, versus sitting outside under a tree. Experience the effect on your body and mind when you're surrounded by nature.

Your body will pick up on the natural frequencies around you: from the sun, to the earth, to the wind, and the living plants and animals that surround you. These are the natural energies human bodies have been immersed in for hundreds of thousands of years; our bodies evolved in harmony with these elements. When you pay attention to how your body feels in nature, I bet you'll be able to feel the difference—and you'll feel better. (Unless you are surrounded by mosquitos, at which point I recom-

---

106 Ibid, Maller.

In this chapter, we'll look at the benefits from specific elements in nature, through sunlight, sleep, grounding, and water, and simple hacks that can help us bring more of these healing elements into our lives.

THE POWER OF LIGHT

Sunlight is necessary: it not only provides fuel for plants through photosynthesis, but it also gives us specific types of energy that are vital for our health. Without the sun, we wouldn't be alive.

In chapter two, we discussed the role of frequency in healing. Sunlight is a wavelength of light and energy, and our bodies are tuned to its frequency. That is why many cultures and religions worship the sun or have sun gods. Through sun exposure on our skin, our bodies produce vital nutrients and hormones, including vitamin D, which is an important component of the immune system. Studies show that getting proper vitamin D from the sun is protective against respiratory infections,[107] without the additional chemicals and toxins one would receive from a flu shot.

Sunlight contains all the wavelengths of light, and different wavelengths create different effects in our bodies. These different light wavelengths can be used for targeted healing hacks.

---

107 Adrian R. Martineau, et al, "Vitamin D Supplementation to Prevent Acute Respiratory Tract Infections: Systematic Review and Meta-Analysis of Individual Participant Data," *BMJ*, 2017.

In our modern lives, where we spend much of our time indoors, we miss out on the full spectrum of light that our bodies are meant to have. Imagine that for years you spend all day indoors exposed to unnatural light frequencies, such as LED light, which lacks frequencies of infrared light that we need, and generates an unnecessary amount of blue light. Too much blue light generates free radicals that are harmful to the eye and health. In addition to artificial light sources, our man-made environments expose us to tons of EMF from WIFI, smart meters, and cell towers. Unnatural EMF is linked to insomnia and proven to cause cancer (we'll dig into the detriments of EMF later in this chapter). Not only that, but our modern processed foods are toxic. What are all these factors a recipe for? Dis-ease. Can you see how the further we are from nature, the sicker we become as a society?

One of the simplest hacks to bring our bodies back to nature is to spend more time in the sun. The pineal gland, known as the "third eye," produces several key hormones in the brain in response to cycles of light and dark. Among these hormones is melanin, the dark pigmentation responsible for tanning after exposure to the sun, which in turn provides more protection from skin damage. The darker the pigmentation of the skin, the better protection you have against DNA damage and folate depletion. Melanin assists in absorbing the right amounts of UV radiation. The darker your skin is and the lower levels of sunlight available where you live, the higher the chances of having low vitamin D. Low vitamin D levels spell dis-ease for the bones, immunity, and overall health.

But how much sunlight is needed? While sunlight is incredibly healing, it can also cause damage in the form of sunburns. Sunlight, like everything else, must be taken in moderation.

As with any of the hacks in this book, pay attention to your body as you spend time in the sun and be sure to protect your skin when you're receiving too much sun. It is important to note that most sunblock is loaded with cancer-causing chemicals and prevents the absorption of nutrients from the sun. If I know I will be out in the sun for a long period of time, I use coconut oil mixed with a tiny bit of zinc, or a really good natural sunblock like Badger Organic Sunscreen, which is usually a mix of oils with natural SPF. For short durations in the sun, coconut oil has enough SPF to protect me from the harmful rays in sunlight and allows me to soak up the good stuff.

"A growing number of scientists are concerned that efforts to protect the public from excessive UVR exposure may be eclipsing recent research demonstrating the diverse health-promoting benefits of UVR exposure," according to a research article titled, "Benefits of Sunlight: A Bright Spot in Human Health." Researchers noted: "Some argue that the health benefits of UVB radiation seem to outweigh the adverse effects, and that the risks can be minimized by carefully managing UVR exposure (e.g., by avoiding sunburn), as well as by increasing one's intake of dietary antioxidants and limiting dietary fat and caloric intake."[108] Think back to the concept of hormesis: a small amount of radiation from the sun may actually be beneficial, but it's all in the dosage.

CHROMOTHERAPY

In addition to infrared, the sauna I use also has medical grade chromotherapy, which gives off different colors from the light

---

108 Ibid, Mead

spectrum that are proven to prevent numerous diseases.[109] Chromotherapy is also known as "color therapy."

A research article on this topic titled "A Critical Analysis of Chromotherapy and Its Scientific Evolution" describes why our bodies benefit from different colors of light:

> Every creature is engulfed in light that affects its health conditions. The human body, according to the doctrine of chromotherapy, is basically composed of colors. The body comes into existence from colors, the body is stimulated by colors, and colors are responsible for the correct working of various systems that function in the body. All organs and limbs of the body have their own distinct color. All organs, cells, and atoms exist as energy, and each form has its frequency or vibrational energy. Each of our organs and energy centers vibrates and harmonizes with the frequencies of these colors. When various parts of the body deviate from these expected normal vibrations, one can assume that the body is either diseased or at least not functioning properly. The vibratory rates inherent in the vibrational technique (chromotherapy) are such that they balance the diseased energy pattern found in the body. For in every organ there is an energetic level at which the organ functions best. Any departure from that vibratory rate results in pathology, whereas restoring the appropriate energy levels to the physical organs results in a healed body.[110]

109 Samina T. Yousuf Azeemi and S. Mohsin Raza, "A Critical Analysis of Chromotherapy and Its Scientific Evolution," *Evidence-Based Complementary and Alternative Medicine*, December 2005, 2(4): 481-488.

110 Ibid, Azeemi

PHOTON THERAPY

Photon therapy, like the kind used in the BioCharger, is also helpful for cellular health. It can stimulate mitochondria and charge up the battery pack of the cell. The waves used in photon therapy are capable of penetrating deep into tissues to rejuvenate dysfunctional cells.

HEALING WITH HEAT

When I was a kid, my family would go to a ski resort that had a hot tub open in the winter. We kids would run up the ski slope in our shorts, make snow angels in the snow, and run back down to sit in the hot tub. At the time, I just did it because I liked the feeling—but as it turns out, this kind of hot/cold contrast is great for the brain and body. Turkish and Korean spas often have cold and hot plunge baths, and the contrast between them creates contraction and expansion of cells and blood vessels, which strengthens arteries and helps with the integrity of the blood brain barrier (especially if you dunk your head under).

There are few ways that you can use contrast to your benefit. The most basic is to take hot and cold showers, turning each on for thirty to sixty seconds. You can also contrast a sauna with cold weather, a cold shower, or an ice bath. I have an ice bath in my back yard, and one of my favorite practices is to get in the ice bath on a hot day, and then lay on a towel on the driveway, where I soak up the energy from the hot pavement.

SAUNAS

Over the past few decades, there have been numerous compelling studies that suggest sauna bathing improves overall health. In the studies, frequent sauna use was associated with a 50 percent lower risk for fatal heart disease, 60 percent lower risk for sudden cardiac death, 51 percent lower risk for stroke, and 46 percent lower risk for hypertension. A famous biohacker, Dr. Ronda Patrick, argues that you, and everyone you care about, should be sitting in a "hot box" for twenty minutes at least a couple of times a week.[111]

The reason saunas are so beneficial for the heart is because they train the vascular system in the same way that physical exercise does. To facilitate sweating, 50 to 70 percent of the blood flows from the core to the skin during a sauna session. The heart rate increases to around 150 beats per minute, and after sauna use, blood pressure and resting heart rate return to a lower baseline.[112]

Our bodies create protective adaptive responses to heat stress, and sauna sessions cause an increase in heat shock proteins, which are associated with longevity and lower age-related disease risk: people who used the sauna two to three times per week had 24 percent lower rates of all-cause mortality[113] and 20 percent lower rates of Alzheimer's. For those who used the sauna four to seven times per week, all-cause mortality was lowered 40 percent, while the risk of Alzheimer's dropped 60 percent. Frequent sauna bathing is also associ-

111 Rhonda Patrick, "Sauna Use as an Exercise Mimetic for Heart and Healthspan," *Found My Fitness,* September 10, 2019.

112 "Scientists Uncover Why Sauna Bathing Is Good for Your Health," *Science Daily,* January 5, 2018.

113 T. Laukkanen, et al, "Association Between Sauna Bathing and Fatal Cardiovascular and All-Cause Mortality Events," *JAMA Internal Medicine,* April 2015, 175(4): 542-548.

ated with lower rates of dementia,[114] and stroke,[115] as well as lower systemic inflammation.[116]

INFRARED SAUNAS

Different frequencies of infrared light have different effects on the body. Near-infrared helps with skin rejuvenation, pain relief, wound healing, and improved immune system. In one study, near-infrared was successfully used to treat tissues stressed by hypoxia, genetic mutation, toxins, and mitochondrial dysfunction.[117] Mid-infrared improves circulation and helps with weight loss and pain relief. Far-infrared also assists in weight loss, as well as helping reduce blood pressure and stimulate detoxification, relaxation, and pain relief. A full-spectrum infrared sauna delivers the benefits of each of these infrared frequencies.

Infrared saunas have a profoundly relaxing effect. When you're in an infrared sauna, you have an opportunity to sit with yourself and your feelings, and while soaking up the light waves, you can also disconnect from the outside world and meditate.

It's important to choose an infrared sauna with low electromagnetic frequency (EMF); if the sauna has high EMF

---

114 "Frequent Sauna Bathing May Protect Men Against Dementia, Finnish Study Suggests," *Science Daily*, December 16, 2016.

115 "Frequent Sauna Bathing Reduces Risk of Stroke," *Science Daily*, May 3, 2018.

116 J. A. Laukkanen and T. Laukkanen, "Sauna Bathing and Systemic Inflammation," *European Journal of Epidemiology*, March 2018, 33(3): 351-353.

117 D. M. Johnstone, et al, "Turning On Lights to Stop Neurodegeneration: The Potential of Near Infrared Light Therapy in Alzheimer's and Parkinson's Disease," *Frontiers of Neuroscience*, January 11, 2016.

radiation, it can be equivalent to stepping into a microwave. The best infrared saunas advertise a low EMF frequency.

The benefits from infrared sauna are numerous and varied and the studies have shown that it can help people with a variety of conditions including cardiovascular disease, congestive heart failure, high blood pressure, arthritis, chronic joint and muscle pain, chronic fatigue, poor digestion, depression, and even diabetes.

HEALING IN OUR SLEEP

Just as we need the light, we also need the darkness. We rely on cycles of light and dark to trigger our natural cycles of wakefulness and rest. We need darkness to bring on the greatest of all healers: sleep.

Sleep is one of the most important things anyone can do for recovery. Throughout this book, we've talked about hacking healing with meditation, breathing, exercise, diet, and cleansing—but sleep trumps them all.

Both sun exposure and deep sleep are not only important for health; they are interrelated. In addition to producing melanin in response to sunlight, the pineal gland also produces an important hormone for sleep: melatonin. The pineal gland is like the brain's radio receiver for frequencies, and it sets the pace for your circadian rhythm. Its operations are highly influenced by our environmental exposure to light and dark.

Melatonin production starts when the sun goes down, or when the eyes are no longer exposed to light, and production stops when there is optic exposure to light. In addition to photoreceptors in our eyes that pick up shifts in the light spectrum, we also have biogenic magnetite in our brains that sense shifts in the earth's electromagnetic field. This is why sleep hygiene is important to pay attention to; today's modern conveniences disrupt our natural cycles. Melatonin is one of the most powerful antioxidants, and according to *Current Opinion in Investigational Drugs May 2006 Review*, it plays a key role in countering cancer, autoimmunity, inflammation, and other infections.[118]

Exposure to bright morning light will cause melatonin to produce earlier in the evening, therefore allowing your body to enter into sleep much easier at night. Melatonin production changes with the seasons as light exposure changes. It's possible to supplement natural bright morning light with artificial light, which has proven to be an effective treatment for seasonal affective disorder (SAD), premenstrual syndrome, and even insomnia. Melatonin has also shown to suppress UVR skin damage.[119]

The reason sunlight can help treat SAD is because melatonin is a precursor to serotonin, the "happy chemical." High serotonin levels are associated with increased happiness and improved mental focus.

In modern life, we spend most of our day indoors, resulting in poor melatonin production, which impacts our lives dramatically. So, if you work indoors and you are looking to heal, it is super important for you to take ten to fifteen minutes outside (with no sunglasses). The sunlight we get

---

118 "Current Opinion in Investigational Drugs," *Thomson Reuters*, May 2006.

119 M. Nathaniel Mead, "Benefits of Sunlight: A Bright Spot for Human Health," *Environmental Health Perspectives*, April 2008, 166(4).

from outside can be 1,000 times greater than the light we get indoors, according to melatonin researcher Russel J. Reiter of the University of Texas Health Science Center.[120] Sunglasses limit the access to sunlight, which changes the rhythms of melatonin production. The argument can easily be made that staying indoors all day, wearing sunglasses all the time, or constantly lathering on toxic sunscreen increases the risk of disease and certain cancers.

Our natural, circadian rhythm gets interrupted by a number of factors as we become disconnected from nature. The blue light of our screens, for example, has a big impact on our natural sleep cycles. When we look at a screen before bed, the blue light sends a message to our brain that it's still daylight out; the brain is stimulated into activity rather than releasing the melatonin we need to fall asleep. New research has shown that LED lights, which have more blue light, may double the risk of cancer because of their effect on our circadian rhythms.[121]

To help yourself get into deep, restorative REM sleep, it's important to practice good sleep hygiene. One of the first steps for good sleep hygiene is to reduce the amount of artificial light you get after dark. I take a walk every evening as it gets dark out, which is a great way for the body to experience the transition from day to night and prepare for sleep. Dim the lights in your house so that your brain isn't reactivated by an onslaught of light. You can also get blue-blocking glasses that filter the blue light out from screens. Lastly, about an

---

120 Ibid, Mead

121 Henry Bodkin, "New LED Streetlights May Double Cancer Risk, New Research Warns," *The Telegraph*, April 26, 2018.

hour before bed, shut off all screens, pick up a book, and read. Reading helps calm the body and prepare you for sleep.

Another common way we disrupt our natural circadian rhythms is by drinking coffee. Consuming caffeine in the morning can have lasting effects throughout the day, and drinking caffeine after 2 p.m. is almost guaranteed to keep your brain active by the time you're going to sleep.[122] If you're trying to get better sleep and you can't let go of your coffee, try to have it as early in the morning as you can, so that you're not drinking caffeine later in the day.

Stephen Cherniske, nutritional biochemist and author of *Caffeine Blues,* describes how caffeine not only disrupts sleep but increases the risk of dozens of disorders, from osteoporosis and diabetes to hypertension and heartburn.[123] Coffee crops are sprayed heavily with pesticides, which not only pose health risks for consumers but for agricultural workers as well. Outside of individual health concerns, caffeine addiction creates environmental impact; acres of rainforest have been destroyed to clear more land for coffee crops.

You can't fuel your life on coffee and expect to get away with it forever; it will catch up to you in one way or another; if you find it's difficult to give up coffee throughout the day, look to the reasons behind your habit. Are you medicating yourself? Are you inspired by what you're doing each day? Are you overworking yourself? You may find it easier to give up caffeine after you've examined what in your life gives you natural energy not artificial energy.

---

122 Frances O'Calaghan, Olav Muurlink, and Natasha Reid, "Effects of Caffeine on Sleep Quality and Daytime Functioning," *Risk Management and Healthcare Policy,* 2018, 11: 263-271.

123 Stephen Cherniske, *Caffeine Blues,* New York: Warner Books, 1998.

As we've mentioned previously, alcohol disrupts sleep, and it's also a nervous system depressant that numbs and disconnects you from the natural signals of your body. If you're drinking alcohol every night before you go to sleep, you're missing out on the natural neurochemicals that get released during deep REM sleep and help reduce stress and inflammation.

Certain natural herbs, minerals, and amino acids, like lemon balm and valerian root, L-theanine, magnesium, and selenium are nervous system calmers that help induce sleep. They can be helpful supplements to take if your body needs a little help preparing for sleep.

Melatonin is also commonly used for sleep, but it's important to note that melatonin is a hormone: any time you take a supplement that replaces a natural hormone, your body will have an adaptive response. This means that if you take melatonin, your body will compensate by releasing less of your natural hormone into the brain. It's always a better route to practice good sleep hygiene to help your body release melatonin naturally, rather than taking a supplement.

That said, there are certain specific cases where this particular hack can be useful. For example, if you're flying around the world and you know you're going to have jet lag, taking a tiny bit of melatonin before sleep will help your body get back onto a circadian rhythm. Wearing blue-blocking glasses while looking at screens can also help. Dave Asprey, founder of Bulletproof 360, has a ton of great hacks on the subject of travel and sleep, which can be found online.

THE BEST TIME FOR SLEEP

Miguel Bethelery notes that in Chinese medicine, every hour of sleep you get before midnight is considered to be worth double the sleep you get from each hour after.[124] If you go to bed at nine and sleep for three hours before midnight, you'll actually need less sleep because the early hours of sleep are more restorative. Someone who goes to bed early may only need six or seven hours of sleep per night, while other people need eight to ten.

We're meant to go to sleep shortly after it gets dark out, but in modern life we often don't. With artificial lights, work, and TV, many people stay up later, and our brains are more stimulated after dark. Not only does this affect the quality of our sleep and the ability to get into deep restorative sleep, but it affects the total number of hours we get. The next day, we're roused by an alarm or the sun or a natural time that the body consistently wakes up, and sometimes that means we haven't gotten the sleep we need.

Sleep was a major factor in my own health challenges. As a personal trainer and the owner of a training facility, I wake up at four in the morning—that's the nature of the profession—and it was only until a few years ago that I started to put sleep hygiene practices into place and take my own sleep seriously. Once I did, it became one of the most profound factors in my healing along with breathwork. Sleep is the body's primary opportunity to repair our systems, reduce inflammation, and relieve stress. Of all of the healing processes presented in this book, sleep is the first priority to work on.

---

124 Miguel Bethelery, in conversation with the author, January 10, 2019.

CONNECT WITH THE GROUND

Another simple and easy technique for stimulating the healing process and bringing the body back to nature is to connect with the earth beneath our feet. All of the atoms of our bodies carry an electrical charge that interacts with the environment around us. Our atoms are constantly exchanging electrons with everything we come into contact with.

There are always ions in the atmosphere around us, and they can take electrons from us, or they can be electron donors. These ions are, on a basic level, exchanging energy with us. As environmental conditions change, they have an effect on us, including on our emotions. When it's very windy, for example, we can tend to feel fatigued much faster because there are lower numbers of ions in the environment exchanging electrons with our bodies.[125] I see this effect with my five-year-old son and his schoolmates: when it's windy and overcast outside and I go pick him up, my son is cranky—the teachers tell me the kids all can get that way from the weather.

Grounding—literally bringing our bodies in direct contact with the ground—is a great way to bring equilibrium back to this electron exchange and bring our bodies back into harmony and connection with the earth. We can do this simply by stepping on the earth in our bare feet.

I remember hearing a story about a man who visited the home of an indigenous American Indian family. The mother looked at the shoes on the man's feet and said, "You shouldn't wear those; they will make you sick." Science is finally catching up with what people have known for thousands of years.

---

125 Walter Sullivan, "Ions Created by Winds May Prompt Changes in Emotional States," *The New York Times*, October 6, 1981.

When we make direct contact with the ground, without the rubber soles of our shoes or concrete and asphalt to insulate us, we exchange electrons directly with the earth and get a donation of antioxidants.

Researchers at the HeartMath Institute found that, "The earth and ionosphere generate a symphony of frequencies ranging from 0.01 hertz to 300 hertz, and some of the large resonances occurring in the earth's field are in the same frequency range as those occurring in the human cardiovascular system, brain, and autonomic nervous system."[126] Our connection with nature helps us tap into the frequencies of nature, and our bodies balance our own frequency and energy in response.

Pulsed electromagnetic field (PEMF) therapy can create similar effects with grounding frequencies. These frequencies are vibrating at the same frequencies of the earth, and they are designed to target the frequencies certain tissues need to re-ionize and rebalance the cells. If you're not able to spend adequate time in nature and soak up the frequencies that keep your body in balance, PEMF therapy can help stimulate healing in cells.

GET IN THE FLOW

When you're exposed to depleting environments that have high positive ions, such as a windy day or exposure to too much WIFI, you can reverse the effects by going into an environment with high negative ions. Waterfalls have high

---

126 "Global Coherence Research," *HeartMath Institute,* 2019.

negative ions; being in clean rivers or in the ocean can bring equilibrium to atoms and calm to our bodies.

Water that contains high negative ions that is coming untainted from Mother Earth is harmonizing and healing. When we spend time in water, we get electrons donated back to our bodies, and we recharge our cells. At my treehouse in Costa Rica, we go the waterfalls and rivers to swim, and after spending time in water, everyone describes feeling rejuvenated and revitalized.

THE IMPORTANCE OF HYDRATION

Our bodies are around 75 percent water, and we're constantly drinking water to replenish our cells. Water is the carrier that brings nutrients into each cell, and it flushes wastes and toxins out. When we're dehydrated, our cells suffer: toxins build up, and inflammation sets in. Drinking plenty of clean water is one of the most important things we can do every day to help our bodies perform at their best.

The sources of our water aren't always pristine, though. Municipal water often has fluoride and chlorine in it, among other chemicals that not only kill pathogens but also kill good gut bacteria and are toxic in the body. An April 2019 study by the Environmental Working Group estimated that contaminants in California's public water systems, including arsenic, hexavalent chromium, and even uranium and radium could have contributed to roughly 15,000 cancer cases in the state.[127] These additives and toxins can damage cells and lower our energy, and it's important to have a good

127 "Study: Up to 15,000 Cancer Cases Could Stem from Chemicals in California Tap Water," *Fox 5 News*, April 29, 2019.

water filter. But think back to Dr. Emoto's work on the power of our thoughts and words: he took samples from a polluted water source and had people pray over the water. When he froze the water that had been prayed over, the resulting ice crystals became beautiful structures.

Some people have a tendency to feel stressed about the toxins in their environment and in their water, but Dr. Emoto's work shows us that our thoughts are powerful. We can send positive energy to the sources of our water and our food, through prayer or positive thoughts, and influence the benefits they hold for our bodies.

UNNATURAL FREQUENCIES

Our manmade environments insulate and disconnect us from the frequencies of nature, and they also raise the number of frequencies that can be disruptive to our health. One of the biggest culprits present in most modern homes is our WIFI and smart meters.

I had the opportunity to interview an expert in the field, James Finn who owns Elexana, an EMF health and safety firm in NYC. He came into this industry after suffering from EMF sensitivity.

Finn was a professional musician for about thirty years, and the combination of being in dark studios with little sunlight and lots of electrical equipment resulted in health problems. He had insomnia, gastroesophageal reflux disease, and other symptoms that he eventually traced back to EMF exposure.

Finn recognized that some people are more sensitive to EMF

than others. Using several different devices, Finn can test the voltage on a person's skin to determine whether they are more sensitive to EMF. He has helped many people identify the harmful EMF in their environment and heal from EMF toxicity.

We are electrical beings, so when you're ill, Finn said, it's an electrical issue. It makes sense to look at the electrical environmental factors in the spaces where you spend the most time. In addition, dietary factors play a role: in Finn's experience, people who eat a vegan diet tend to experience more severe symptoms from EMF exposure, perhaps because of the difference in lipids that insulate the nerves and amino acids in the diet.[128]

I noticed in my own healing journey that WIFI had a disruptive effect on my system. Similarly, at our training facility, I noticed that people were coming in with common complaints: they felt dizzy and lethargic, and they reported being distracted by their devices. They were experiencing a lot of headaches. I suspected these were all side effects of unnatural frequencies wreaking havoc on their systems. After researching more and more about the topic, I began to recommend people limit their exposure to WIFI. One of my trainers had a two-month-old baby sleeping next to the WIFI router in their house, and the first night he shut off the WIFI, he said his baby had the best night of sleep he'd had since he was born. In my clients and in myself, I noticed huge improvements in health by taking steps to cut down the WIFI radiation we were exposing ourselves to on a daily basis.

---

128 James Finn, in conversation with the author, August 23, 2019.

Many natural healers will not work with people who don't first make an effort to reduce WIFI exposure, because without reducing the radiation exposure in your home environment, healing is an uphill battle.

You can purchase a Faraday cage to put around your WIFI router, and it will reduce the amount of electromagnetic radiation from your router, while still allowing a signal out to your devices. You can program your router or power circuit to shut off at night when you're not using it.

WIFI is one common source of radiation, but there can also be other electromagnetic frequencies (EMF) in your home that disrupt your cells' healing processes. Studies have shown that people who live near power lines, for example, have higher risk for leukemia and other cancers.[129] Cell phones have also been linked strongly to cancer risk. Laptops emit radiation as well.

There are protective mats, cell phone covers, or clothing pieces you can buy for using your laptop, so that you reduce the amount of radiation you receive from your devices. Some of these products are effective, but many of them are not. The only way to know a genuine product from a scam is to use a device to measure its effectiveness. I use a tri-field meter to test the products I purchase. Make sure to get these products from a trusted source and look for reviews or videos of people who have tested the products to see if they actually work. Use headphones when talking on your cell phone to create more distance from your device.

---

129 Daniel J. DeNoon, "Child Leukemia Again Linked to Power Lines," *Chronic Lymphocytic Leukemia*, June 2, 2005.

If you're chronically ill, it's a good idea to test your home for EMF levels. Smart meters are constantly emitting high levels of radiation, and increase the amount of EMF in the home. You can buy a tri-field meter or hire an expert to test your EMF exposure from your WIFI and other sources of radiation in your house, such as from smart meters or cell towers.

Frequent air travel also exposes us to unnatural frequencies, both through the body-imaging machines used at TSA checkpoints (which have been shown to shed DNA), and through the WIFI in the plane, which is trapped in the aluminum aircraft. We can compensate for this radiation in two ways. First, you can reduce your exposure to it by wearing radiation-blocking clothing when you travel. Second, you can give a boost to your cells by supplementing with vitamin C and magnesium. Your nutrition can help mitigate the effect of the radiation your body receives.

CHANGE YOUR ENVIRONMENT

We are all impacted by our environment. Often in modern life, the environments we choose to live in cause us to disconnect from nature. We spend our time walking on concrete instead of the ground, and we light our lives with lightbulbs instead of the sun. We trade the frequencies of the natural world for the frequency of WIFI. In turn, these environmental factors influence our emotions, thoughts, and ultimately, our beliefs. In chapter two, we discussed the importance of our thoughts and beliefs in influencing the journey to health, and one powerful way to reset our thoughts and beliefs is to reset our environment.

When I do retreats in Costa Rica, one of the biggest benefits is that the retreat setting takes people out of their normal environment. When we remove ourselves from the environment we're always in, we can show up differently. Often, people will arrive on day one with the stress and constricted beliefs and view of their old environment, but shortly into the retreat, they realize they have different thoughts, and feelings that produce different actions, interactions, and revelations. They let go. The natural environment transforms people and opens the space for them to find their soul's calling, which is what life is all about.

On the last retreat I hosted at the treehouse, we had an eighteen-year-old kid in the program who'd come with his father. His mom told me that before the retreat, he was uncommunicative and distant, and he wouldn't come out of his room. After the retreat, he was engaging with his family, reading more in shared family spaces, and communicating in ways he hadn't before.

Such a huge transformation comes from the change in environment and the change in daily practices that we did together on the retreat, such as connecting with the natural environment around us, taking in more oxygen with breathwork, doing ice baths, and eating organic food grown right on the property. Throughout, we work on identifying our stories and beliefs that don't serve us and tap into what gives us inspiration. When this eighteen-year-old returned home, he was more in touch with his body and his soul's calling. He was a talented artist and started drawing again. When people have more clarity, more direction, more truth, more love, more energy, and more connection to source, they are elevated to heights that they never even knew existed.

Many people die never knowing that life can be filled with

such serenity, peace, and joy. These effects are common on our retreat. But many of these benefits are not just isolated to a Costa Rican treehouse, of course; taking a trip to any natural environment can help open you up to new experiences and perspectives. The beach is one of the best environments to relieve stress, research shows, because it combines the effects of the elements we've discussed in this chapter. The rhythmic sound of the waves can put us into a meditative state, while the light has a calming effect on the brain. Ocean air contains negative ions that have a positive effect on your mood, and walking barefoot in the sand grounds your body.[130]

When you pay attention to and provide for your body's needs, connect with nature, and open your mind to new thoughts, transformation can occur.

THE HACKS

Accessible Methods
- Spend the right amount of time in the sun to boost your immune system, sleep patterns, vibration, and your vitamin D.
- Spend time in clean rivers with water falls to re-ionize and recharge your cells.
- Sit in a sauna a few times a week.
- Walk barefoot on the ground.
- Practice good sleep hygiene by dimming lights after dark and reading for an hour before bedtime and wear blue-blocking glasses after sundown.

---

130 Anne Gherini, "Recent Studies Show that the Beach is One of the Best Places to Alleviate Stress and Heal Your Brain," *Inc.*, November 20, 2017.

Advanced Methods
- Nature retreats.
- Pulsed Electromagnetic Field (PEMF) therapy (the BioCharger, AmpCoil, and Bemer are a few devices I have used).
- Infrared saunas.

Things to Consider Avoiding
- Consider keeping WIFI off as much as possible; set a timer on your router to turn off WIFI during the hours it's not in use.
- Beware of the increased EMF you receive while traveling; wear radiation-blocking clothing and increase antioxidants: take vitamin C (stay away from GMO corn-based supplements) and magnesium supplements to mitigate the effects.

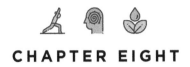

CHAPTER EIGHT

CARVING NEW PATHWAYS WITH PSYCHEDELICS

Stanislav Grof, a Czech psychiatrist and creator of holotropic breathwork, began working with LSD after his first session with the medicine in 1956. During his session, he had a doctor measure his brain activity with EEG while also stimulating the brain with stroboscopic light. Throughout the trip, the doctor adjusted the stroboscopic light to create alpha, theta, and delta waves in Grof's brain. The results were profound. "My consciousness was catapulted out of my body," he said of the experience. "I became all of existence."[131]

When the light was shut off, Grof reported that the world started "shrinking" again, and he had a hard time aligning his consciousness back with his body. From this experience, Grof concluded that consciousness is cosmic, and the brain is only a moderator of consciousness. Grof went on to study psychedelics and states of consciousness for six decades, sitting in on around 4,500 LSD sessions. He predicted that LSD will do for psychiatry what the microscope did for biology.

---

131 "Stan Grof—Lessons from ~4,500 LSD Sessions and Beyond," *The Tim Ferris Show*, December 13, 2018.

Today, there is still a lot of stigma and misconception around psychedelics, but it is important to know that their therapeutic effects have been researched for decades (and in some indigenous communities, for generations). There are many different kinds of psychedelics, including LSD, San Pedro, ibogaine, psilocybin (mushrooms), ayahuasca, and peyote, and they all have different therapeutic effects. This chapter is devoted to these medicines, which have had a profound effect on my own healing.

The first time I took a legal therapeutic microdose of psilocybin, I felt my cells begin to vibrate. Throughout my health challenges, certain cells in my body have become like barometers or tuning forks, and as I've worked to heal certain areas of my body, I've been able to feel changes down to the cellular level. For example, if I hold a crystal rock up to my jaw, the cells in my jaw will start vibrating, and my jaw begins to visibly shake. Every time I show this trick to someone in my family, they're weirded out by the effect. This sensitivity is what has made my health experiments so powerful: I can feel the frequency and energy of most things instantly. The first time I microdosed with psilocybin, I felt an immediate shift. I knew this was medicine—and a powerful one at that.

In addition to the systemic health issues I was sorting out leading up to taking psilocybin, I had also been experiencing numbness, like a neuropathy, down one arm and leg (as a residual effect of improper detox method). As soon as the dose kicked in, I started to feel a vibration radiating through those areas of my body. It's difficult to describe what the experience felt like and probably even more difficult for the people to whom I've described it to truly understand, except to say that I felt my cells waking up. The numbness in my arm and leg dissipated, along with the tension I'd been holding in my jaw. It was like the mushroom was eating up the toxins in my body. Even though the dose I'd taken was very small, I could feel it creating an incredible effect in my body. More important than the sensations I felt during the experience was the effect I felt after. My mood improved, and I felt far less reactive to stress. Plant medicine, for me, has been powerful medicine.

Of course, not everyone agrees. The Food and Drug Administration (FDA) classifies psilocybin, alongside other psychedelic medicines, as Schedule I controlled substances. Schedule I substances are deemed to have no accepted medical benefit, in addition to a high potential for abuse. The FDA's Schedule I list includes marijuana, LSD, and heroin. Schedule II controlled substances are considered to have medical benefit but a high risk of dependence. Many narcotics are in this category. Schedule III includes drugs with a moderate risk of dependence, and Schedule IV includes many prescription drugs, from sleep medications to anti-anxiety drugs, that have a low potential for abuse.

According to the FDA, psilocybin is up there with the worst offenders in terms of safety, and it's illegal in the US. But for the past twenty years, the John Hopkins University Psychedelic Research Unit has been exploring the effects and benefits of psilocybin on mental health conditions. Their studies have led researchers to advocate for changing the classification of psilocybin from Schedule I to Schedule IV, so that it can be used like other prescription drugs for the benefit of patients.[132]

132 Peter Hess, "Magic Mushrooms Should Be Less Illegal, Scientists Argue," *Inverse*, September 27, 2018.

I decided to experiment with these medicines legally in part because I'd already seen what pharmaceutical drugs had done. Some of the drugs I'd been given in hospitals and prescribed by doctors had negative impacts on my mind and my overall health. The amalgam fillings, Accutane, Concerta, Wellbutrin, Paxil, Zoloft, vaccines, and fluoroquinolone antibiotics all had devastating long-term effects on my body. If these FDA-approved drugs, which had been formulated and synthesized in a lab, could be so detrimental to me, did I really trust what the FDA had to say about a plant medicine that came from the earth? The research I'd found, including studies from Johns Hopkins, pointed to the positive potential this medicine could have for someone like me, who was dealing with neurological issues and depressive symptoms.

Johns Hopkins researchers have been doing guided therapeutic psilocybin sessions for people with anxiety, depression, alcoholism, addiction, and post-traumatic stress disorder, and their results are profound. In one study, 70 percent of the participants reported that their psilocybin session was among the top five most meaningful experiences of their lives; 83 percent said it was among the top five most significant spiritual experiences of their lives; and 94 percent reported an increased sense of wellbeing or life satisfaction after the session.[133] Participants described having an increased sense of personal authenticity, playfulness, creativity, mental flexibility, and self-confidence. They had an increased appreciation and sense of meaning in their lives. These experiences didn't just affect participants' feelings; 89 percent said they also experienced positive behavior changes after their psilocybin sessions.

---

133 "Hallucinogenic Drug Psilocybin Eases Existential Anxiety in People with Life-Threatening Cancer," *Johns Hopkins Medicine*, December 1, 2016.

In part due to a push from the Johns Hopkins studies, laws are shifting around these substances, as well. As of this writing, the city of Denver became the first to decriminalize psilocybin. Given the strong research backing the therapeutic effects of psilocybin, this may be the first step of many to change the legal standing of these medicines. Researchers in New Zealand are preparing to launch the first-ever clinical trials of microdosing for LSD and psilocybin.[134] Other groups are dedicated to researching MDMA, ketamine, and LSD for their therapeutic effects. And in September of 2019, Johns Hopkins opened the Center for Psychedelics and Conscious Research to investigate psychedelic treatments for issues like depression, smoking, alcoholism, anorexia, Lyme disease, Alzheimer's, and opioid addiction.[135]

REWIRING TRAUMA

The Johns Hopkins researchers concluded that one of the reasons psychedelics like psilocybin are so effective is that they stimulate our bodies to repair neurons in our brains. One explanation for certain mental health conditions, such as depression, is that they stem from damaged neural pathways, particularly in the prefrontal cortex.

Until recently, it was thought that by the age of thirty, your neural connections were set; your brain would function the same way from then on, with the same thought patterns. Any damage that occurred to brain cells at that point was

---

134 Randy Robinson, "The World's First Clinical Trials on Microdosing LSD and Psilocybin Are Coming," *Merry Jane*, August 20, 2019.

135 Jean Lotus, "Psychedelic Drug Therapy Enters a New Era with Johns Hopkins Center," *United Press International*, September 27, 2019.

thought to be permanent, because after a certain age brain cells couldn't regenerate.

We now know that's not true. Throughout our lives, our brains are capable of repairing neural connections, and growing new neurons. Neurogenesis, or the creation of new neurons, is stimulated by many factors, including endurance exercise.[136] And, we now know, psychedelics can also trigger the brain to heal and repair.

Psychedelics can induce *neuroplasticity*, encouraging the growth and connection of new neurons, to rewire those connections on a cellular level.[137]

In chapter two, we looked at the progression for how our thoughts and feelings become beliefs. Many of our beliefs are laid down in early childhood, from ages one to seven. At those early ages, we develop negative and positive associations with the world around us. These associations, in turn, carve pathways in our brains, and create our reactions to similar stimuli in the future. Someone who has a phobia of spiders, for example, has a pathway built into their neurons: the sight of a spider triggers an automatic fight-or-flight response in the brain.

It's possible to shift these pathways through repetition of positive thoughts and associations. The daily dozen gratitude practice and the golden light meditation described earlier can both reinforce positive networks in the brain with con-

---

136 "Sustained Aerobic Exercise Increases Adult Neurogenesis in Brain," *Science Daily*, February 8, 2016.

137 Peter Hess, "Psychedelic Drugs Reshape Cells to "Repair" Neurons in Our Brains," *Inverse*, June 13, 2018.

sistent practice. The more often you bring gratitude into your awareness, the more fully you feel it.

Psychedelics fast-track and enhance that work by breaking up negative pathways. Neuroimaging studies have even produced images of the changes to the structures of dendrites and nerves as a result of psychedelic therapies.[138] These medicines can act as a neural reset, opening up the possibility for us to create new thought patterns, stories, and belief systems. These effects have been studied in psilocybin, LSD, 5-MEO-DMT, and ayahuasca.

The compounds in psilocybin in particular have the ability to counteract structural and functional issues in the brain, including combatting depression.[139] A 2018 study also showed that microdosing on psychedelics gave people a boost in creativity and open-mindedness.[140] Personality changes can be lasting: in a one-year follow-up of one study, participants were still one standard deviation higher in metrics of openness—signaling a profound shift.

Malin Uthaug, a PhD graduate at Maastricht University in Prague in ayahuasca and 5-meo-DMT, researches the effect of psychedelics on mental health. I had the opportunity to interview her during the final stages of her PhD in Prague shortly after my Wim Hof Master certification in Poland. She said that people with certain mental health conditions,

---

138 Calvin Ly, et al, "Psychedelics Promote Structural and Functional Neuro Plasticity," *Cell Replication*, June 12, 2018, 23(11): 3170-82.

139 Jesse Hicks, "Active Ingredient in Shrooms Could 'Reset' Brains of Depressed People," *Vice*, October 13, 2017.

140 Thomas Anderson and Rotem Petranker, "Microdosing on LSD May Make You Wiser and More Creative, Study Reveals," *Inverse*, November 6, 2018.

such as PTSD, "Tend to just focus on their problem inside this box. Ayahuasca allows you to start thinking outside of the box, away from that problem."

She described how typically we solve problems in life with the same kind of "convergent thinking" we use to solve math problems. Uthaug said, "With convergent thinking, there's only one solution. Someone with the pressure of PTSD is just banging their head against the wall, trying to solve that problem with only one way." But an ayahuasca trip increases our divergent thinking. "You can look at things from a different angle and perhaps come up with a better way of tackling the problem."[141]

YOUR INTENTIONS SHAPE YOUR BRAIN

When using psychedelics (or doing anything that matters in life), it is important to look at the "set and setting."

"Set and setting" refers to the conditions of your session. This includes the physical and social environment you're in, as well as your mental and emotional state. Where do you plan to take the medicine, and who do you plan to take it with?

It could be said that your intention for every action will determine whether you heal or not. Your intention and where you focus your attention may be the most important factors for your health.

The HeartMath Institute describes it this way:

---

141 Malin Uthaug, in conversation with the author, December 6, 2018.

When we activate the power of our hearts' commitment and intentionally have sincere feelings such as appreciation, care and love, we allow our hearts' electrical energy to work for us...Consciously choosing a core heart feeling over a negative one means instead of the drain and damage stress causes to our bodies' systems, we are renewed mentally, physically, and emotionally. The more we do this, the better we're able to ward off stress and energy drains in the future. Heartfelt positive feelings fortify our energy systems and nourish the body at the cellular level. At HeartMath, we call these emotions quantum nutrients.[142]

In a conversation with my friend Diane Kazer, we discussed the concept that "you are the supplement"—meaning that your thoughts and feelings trigger the chemicals the body needs to naturally heal you in many ways. She told me the story of Robert Richman, who created the "XPill," a placebo pill filled with brown rice powder. Richman put these placebo pills in bottles meant to look like prescription pill bottles, and he took them to Burning Man. Before giving people an XPill, he told them to hold an intention in their mind, and after the pill was taken, people experienced "aha" moments and powerful shifts. A psychologist who learned about the XPill began giving them to her patients, and reported that they had breakthroughs they otherwise hadn't had.

The point is, just setting an intention can lead to massive transformation. Intention is the "set" of set and setting.

With the use of psychedelics, your mind becomes malleable. As old patterns get broken down, your brain is open to new

---

142 "You Can Change Your DNA," *HeartMath*, July 14, 2011.

pathways. In working with these medicines, your intentions, beliefs, and reasons for doing the therapy all have a major impact on your experience and how those neural connections rebuild.

Like many people, I experimented with psychedelics recreationally in my younger years. Some of those times were among the best experiences of my life, and others were scary. My lack of intention resulted in a mixed bag of experiences that was not used for spiritual growth or healing.

When you take psychedelics in environments where you're surrounded by chaos, fear, frustration, and anger, those feelings can be amplified by the medicine. Negative conditions can lead you to not only have a negative experience but to also develop a negative association with what psychedelics are capable of. On the other hand, if you hold your intention toward more love, gratitude, peace, and comfort, you allow those emotions to steer your experience.

You want to create a relaxed environment, and you want the people around you to be those you're emotionally comfortable with. Your mindset is important, too. Don't go into a trip if you're angry, frustrated, and pissed off. Your emotional state will set the tone for your trip.

Set an intention. What do you want to get out of the session? Your intention can guide where the medicine takes you. These are plants that have spirits, and while they're not to be played with, they can be utilized to have profound transformations.

In my experience, I've found it's important to set a positive intention. The medicine can bring up unexpected experiences, and a positive intention helps you approach your trip in a positive light. If you plan to take ayahuasca, for example, and you ask the medicine to start the healing process, that journey may involve aspects that are unpleasant, such as reliving traumatic experiences that have been trapped in your body. The medicine helps release these experiences so they can be processed outside the body, rather than staying stuck in the limbic system, or the fight-or-flight mode of our nervous system. Some people go into a trip asking the medicine to show them fear—and while exploring that intention can be beneficial, it's important to be clear with yourself about why you want to explore that emotion. Often, combat veterans do a lot of purging during ceremonies; guides will say that is the process of anger, fear, and other negative emotions being purged out.

Taking the influence of set and setting into account, the Johns Hopkins researchers had participants listen to a special, seven-hour-long playlist to help with guiding the participant's psilocybin experience. You can look up the Johns Hopkins playlist on Spotify: it includes a series of instrumental pieces and ends with recognizable songs, like hits from the Beatles and Louis Armstrong's "What a Wonderful World." I've used this playlist for my own experiences with megadosing, and found the music took me on a journey and gave me a powerful experience. Remember, music has the ability to light up certain parts of the brain, so certain sounds may trigger certain brainwaves in various centers of the brain.

When you allow your positive belief and your spirit to guide the experience, you also allow those qualities to guide the way your neural connections rebuild. One of the powerful effects of psychedelics is that they help dissolve the ego. New neural connections go on to influence your responses to the world, and therefore your life.

I interviewed Dr. Steve Young, who has been in the health field for over twenty-three years, and he described why intention is so important in taking plant medicines. In the west, he said, we tend to think of these medicines as chemicals that influence our brains. But in other cultures, he said, "It's literally alive. It's a spirit you're working with, not just some inanimate chemical equation. It has its own intentions and intelligence, and you're dancing with this spirit inside you. You want to go into the experience with very high reverence and intention."[143]

This is 100 percent true in my experience. Before my own experiences with plant medicine, I didn't understand what people meant when they referred to the "spirit" of ayahuasca. It's hard for the Western mind to understand this concept, and the best way for me to understand it was through experience. During the time that I was sick, I progressively lost the connection to my spirit. The sicker I became the more disconnected I felt from spirit or God. When I took ayahuasca for the first time, I finally felt a spirit coming back to me, and I reconnected. The medicine is a mirror. It reveals to you what you already know you have within.

The conditions under which you decide to experiment with these medicines, and the environment set up to do so, should be taken very seriously. It's recommended to work with a professional guide to facilitate the experience.

---

143 Steve Young, in conversation with the author, March 22, 2019.

BREAKING CYCLES OF ADDICTION

Some research is now pointing to the ability of psychedelics to break cycles of addiction. A recent study showed that therapeutic sessions with LSD helped with the cessation or reduction of alcohol use disorder.[144]

After I read an article on this study, I posted my thoughts on social media. Soon after, I got a private message from a friend (who is also a Wim Hof instructor) describing how psychedelics had changed his life. He'd had a serious problem with alcohol, he wrote, and for years he'd been unable to stop and couldn't figure out what was going on. He decided to take a high dose of psilocybin to see if the medicine could shift it, and his addiction dissipated. He'd only done one session, and it was years ago, but it had a lasting effect: his addiction had gone away completely, and he hadn't had an issue since.

Because of their ability to break up pathways in our brains, psychedelics can stop addiction dead in its tracks. Two observational studies demonstrated that another psychedelic, ibogaine, had an 80 percent success rate for stopping heroin addiction.[145] I think of the possibilities these medicines could offer to friends I know who have gotten addicted to painkillers and struggled with pharmaceutical treatments like methadone with no relief. Plant medicines are extremely powerful, and because of their criminal classification, most people don't know the potential these medicines have for treating illness and reconnecting people with their true selves.

144 Sarah Sloat, "Psychedelics' Role in Beating Alcoholism Illustrated in LSD, Psilocybin Study," *Inverse*, May 17, 2019.

145 "What Is the Success Rate for Ibogaine?" *American Addiction Centers*, September 3, 2019.

BUILDING NEW CONNECTIONS WITH AYAHUASCA

When people reconnect with themselves, their lives are transformed: I've seen it hundreds of times, and I've experienced it personally. As each of us individually reconnects with our true nature to heal ourselves, we heal the world as well. As Gandhi said, "Be the change you wish to see in the world," because everything is a projection of your own psyche.

In addition to my experiences microdosing and megadosing with psilocybin, I've also experimented with various forms of ayahuasca. During those experiences, I've met practitioners and guides who believe that ayahuasca and other psychedelics are a gift from nature to help the world heal itself.

There are two components of ayahuasca: the vine of the plant is the traditional basis for the ayahuasca brew, while the leaf of the plant contains DMT, which amplifies the effect of the vine to create its psychedelic effects.

I went to a retreat in Peru at the Temple of the Way of the Light to experience an ayahuasca ceremony guided by healers from the Amazon. Guides will tell you that as you become open to the idea of taking ayahuasca, the spirit of the plant will begin to call to you. That was certainly the case for me. I felt the calling to try ayahuasca for five or six years before I finally decided to take part in a ceremony. I encountered mentions of the medicine everywhere, and it was on my radar nonstop. It kept popping up in my life, and everyone I was meeting was telling me about it. I understood what it means for the medicine to call to you. I did tons of research before deciding to commit—probably too much, because given the amount of healing I received in one week, I should have done it years ago.

In preparation for the ceremony, our guides instructed us to do a "dieta." The dieta is a set of restrictions that are recommended before and after an ayahuasca ceremony. For three to four weeks before and after the ceremony, we were told to cut out red meat, pork, alcohol, recreational drugs, masturbation, sex, and other plant medicines. Additionally, we were told to eat a diet of low fat and no salt. These preparations might have been the toughest part of the journey, but not all cultures or places follow these strict measures. The reason behind it is so the body is cleaner to receive the connection with the ayahuasca.

Our guides were members of the Shipibo tribe, and as they served the ayahuasca, they sang what's called the *icaros*, or sacred songs to call the spirit. Often, an ayahuasca ceremony begins with a cleansing song to clear out the negative energies and toxins the participants have been exposed to, and the guide will follow with a song specific to each participant's needs. The guide uses the icaros to communicate with the spirit and modulate the energy of the plant to help the person taking the medicine. In chapter two we looked at the benefits of sound meditation; these healers were using harmony and sound for healing and connecting with the spirits.

Our guides poured the ayahuasca brew into a shot glass for each of the participants. For some of us with specific issues, before we were each given our dose of the brew, one of the *curanderos*, or healers, would hold the shot glass up to his mouth and sing the icaros specific to the issues the person was healing into the ayahuasca before consumption.

The first night I wasn't able to drink the ayahuasca brew with the rest of the participants because I had some serious gut issues happening. But I still sat for the ceremony and I could feel the power of the spirit and the power of the healing songs. Even though I hadn't taken the medicine, I felt the spirit entering my body the first night. I recognized this feeling because I have had it happen to me previously when I was at the lowest point of my health crisis.

My brain and my whole body had been inflamed for a year, and I had the stabbing pain in the back of the head that I've previously described. As a coach, I was an avid researcher of neuroscience and brain health, and I'd picked up a massive brain science book, hoping I would get insights to healing the pain in my head. One night, I came home with my girlfriend after being away all weekend and this book was standing upright, open, in the middle of the floor. I asked my girlfriend if she had moved my brain book, but she said no.

All of a sudden, I felt the spirit come into my body. The spirit massaged my head where the headache was. It reassured me the healing process was starting. Shortly after, my girlfriend asked if I was okay; she sensed something was off. I told her I thought I'd just seen a ghost.

During the ayahuasca ceremony, we were meant to sit upright, so that the crown of our head was reaching up to the sky. This position keeps the spine in alignment and allows the energy to enter the body, but the first night the healing was so profound that I could barely sit up and stay awake.

The next night, because I had some health issues going on at the time, an icaros specific for my healing was sung into my glass of ayahuasca. The curandero took his time, singing the icaros over my shot glass for five to ten minutes and then gave the shot to me.

As the ayahuasca began to work on me, I received a message from myself—or the spirit of the plant, however you want to look at it—saying *we've been waiting for you*. In the first part of the journey, I felt I was being returned back to my true self. The experience was profound and blissful, and it felt like I was exactly where I needed to be.

You will know when you're ready to take ayahuasca: it will be everywhere in your attention. It will call to you. The spirit of the plant begins its work on you long before you take it. After all, it is the process of reconnecting to your true self and expunging all the low-vibrational energy, toxins, and poison that you have accumulated along your life. The expelling of the poisons can be uncomfortable, but everyone I spoke with afterwards said it was a beautiful experience.

LEGAL METHODS FOR PLANT MEDICINES

Most psychedelic substances are illegal in the US. However, there are certain churches that are allowed to use ayahuasca for religious reasons, and you can also travel outside of the US for these experiences.

It's possible to access the benefits of ayahuasca legally with vine-only ayahuasca. Vine-only ayahuasca does not contain DMT found in the leaf, which means it is not psychedelic, therefore it's not a controlled substance. Vine-only ayahuasca can be purchased and taken legally in the US. It contains some of the same benefits for neurogenesis, and it opens new pathways in the brain. One particular healer, Dennis Notten, facilitates vine-only ayahuasca programs in the US, that include intention setting and daily meditations while taking microdoses of vine-only ayahuasca.

While it's illegal to sell or buy psilocybin, it's not illegal to grow the mushrooms. You can buy grow kits online. However, remember that intention and environment are important parts of the healing powers of these medicines: it's crucial to have a professional guide who can help you navigate these experiences for their full healing benefits.

THE IMPORTANCE OF A GUIDE

Psychedelic experiences can be overwhelming, and it's important to have a guide to help you navigate the process and make sure it stays aligned with your intention.

In the Johns Hopkins studies, about 3 percent of the participants who took a high dose of psilocybin experienced anxiety and negative experiences during their sessions. That 3 percent is what the professional is there for: they can ensure that a person who finds themselves sliding into a negative experience can be guided to a place where their experience feels manageable and beneficial.

Just like you would vet a trainer or coach, in looking for a guide or a shaman, you want to find someone who is experienced. Make sure you vet the professionals you choose to work with. You don't want to work with an amateur or a weekend-certification shaman. Ideally you want to work with someone who is indigenous to an area where ayahuasca has been used for thousands of years and who has passed through the cultural training as a healer. If they have no clue how to handle the different effects that these medicines can have, they can make a negative trip even worse. I have heard and read about many instances of people not being prepared enough for what they are getting into, not doing the dietas, not working with someone who knows the true power of these psychedelics—and as a result they don't get the healing they need, or they are left traumatized.

Much of the knowledge around ceremonial plant medicine is passed down generationally, and you can find guides who come from tribes like the Shipibo people, who have long lineages in the work of plant medicine. In Peru, I worked with guides at the Temple of the Way of the Light. They had a rigorous screening process for potential candidates that included questions on psychiatric history, as well as a phone interview to make sure that participants were a good match for their program.

Certain antidepressants such as MAO-inhibitors and other medications cannot be taken with ayahuasca, and an experienced guide will ask thorough questions to make sure the medicine is right for you.

You can also find experienced shamans working in the US. As you look for a guide, be sure to speak with prior attendees of their ceremonies to get a sense of their experience.

THE VIEW FROM THE MOUNTAINTOP

Dennis Notten describes plant medicine ceremonies as

providing a view from the top of a mountain. It allows us a temporary shift in our state of consciousness so that we can have an expansive view: we can see every step that leads us to the mountaintop, and we can see all the potential that results from our journey. As he said in an interview with me, "Now you've thought about it, you've felt it, and then you come out of the ceremony—but you have not lived it."

Plant medicines can create an amazing spark for our next stage of healing, but we have to integrate those experiences with the rest of our lives. We can gain insight and inspiration from these experiences, and then we have to put them into action, with the support of all our healing practices. "The journey of life is to walk that same mountain step by step, breath by breath, sometimes three steps forward and two steps back," Notten said. "You go through all those challenges, all those winding roads in the 3D reality of your life, so you can live that vision."[146]

THE IMPACT OF PLANT MEDICINES

I've been medicinally experimenting with psychedelics for three years, by microdosing and megadosing psilocybin, visiting Peru for ayahuasca ceremonies, and microdosing with vine-only ayahuasca and iboga. In that year, I've seen an increase in my creativity, productivity, and energy. These medicines have reduced my anxiety and improved my mental health and family life. I've even shifted my attitudes around certain beliefs, and I've been able to better focus on the things that truly matter.

---

146 Dennis Notten, in conversation with the author, May 11, 2019.

Most importantly, I relate to people differently and connect more fully with others. Among the multitude of benefits I've experienced from psychedelics, I've noticed that I've increased my capacity to handle stress from my business and my family. Between my EarthFIT facilities and my back-pain program, I'm running four businesses and I have two young kids; my stress levels are high. I come home and instantly have two young kids jumping all over me in a joyful explosion of energy and noise. I used to get frustrated because I couldn't relax. I couldn't tap into that rest and recovery parasympathetic system. For years and years, I was living in fight or flight. I would frequently get angry and have outbursts at my kids or my wife.

While I've been doing a lot of different things to work on these emotional responses, I found the biggest benefit comes from my experiences with psychedelics. I'm no longer as frustrated or as angry. Some people use alcohol or cannabis to create this effect, but those substances tend to repress emotions and keep them from coming to the surface.

Psilocybin and ayahuasca are not like that. Rather than push emotions and experiences down, these medicines allow emotions to come to the surface to be released. They allow us to connect to our true selves—in fact, psychedelics are often called "the connectors." When I practice with these medicines, I ask the plant to show me gratitude, or freedom, or another intention that aligns to a higher vibration I want to access in myself.

When we're more connected to ourselves, we can bring our true selves to others and create deeper connections with the loved ones in our lives.

THE HACKS

Accessible Methods
- Vine-only ayahuasca programs, like those found through Dennis Notten: sacredjourney.earth.
- Psilocybin grow kits.

Advanced Methods
- International travel for psychedelic ceremonies, such as ayahuasca ceremonies found in Peru: templeoft-hewayoflight.org.

Things to Consider Avoiding
- Do not use plant medicines without a guide; the intentions and environments around your experience are crucial for the greatest healing effects.

CONCLUSION

*"We are slowed-down sound and light waves, a walking bundle
of frequencies tuned into the cosmos. We are souls dressed
up in sacred biochemical garments, and our bodies are the
instruments through which our souls play their music."*

—ALBERT EINSTEIN

All the practices and hacks in this book can be summed up
with a simple analogy: Think of yourself as a big battery,
a superconductor, and each of your cells as small batteries. When there is a breakdown in the system, you need a
massive net-positive amount of energy to heal. The hacks
discussed in this book charge your batteries; and when you
understand the influences in your life that drain your battery power, you can reduce your exposure or eliminate those
factors altogether.

Think of earth as the "mother board" designed to support
you. All humans on that mother board are powered by its
magnetic and electric charge. Nature provides free energy,
which is around you all the time, waiting to be soaked up
by you if you are open to it. We all have access to the same
sources that can charge us or deplete our power. Some people
are operating at 10 percent power, while others' batteries are

overflowing. Some actions and feelings charge your battery, and some actions and feelings deplete your battery. Some people drain your battery (energy vampires), while some people recharge your battery. A basic and most simple formula for healing is do more things that charge your battery than deplete your battery.

In this system, you have two features to work with: hardware and software. The hardware is your body, which is an unbelievably beautiful masterpiece of a machine that will work in your favor all day every day if you honor it with things that will nurture it and recharge its batteries. Your hardware was factory installed in your DNA with certain skills, talents, passions, and loves. A bird doesn't need to be shown how to fly, for example; that skill is factory-installed in its DNA. To perform at our best, we have to align our innate hardware with a great software that consistently gets upgraded.

The software is the programming that is running your life: it is your thoughts, feelings, habits, rituals, actions, and environment that are manifesting your experience. Many people are running programs—in the form of their belief systems and stories from media, family, friends, and society—that not only don't serve them but break down the hardware faster and cause dis-ease.

When our hardware and software are working in harmony, we can readily charge our batteries with free energy from nature and the universe. When our hardware or software are out of sync, the system can get bogged down.

Pay attention to the things that deplete your battery, and limit or eliminate these influences in your life:

- Stress on your hardware (your body): too little sleep, not enough water, too much screen time, too much time indoors, excess weight, and too much WIFI exposure.
- Exposure to toxins, including toxic environments, beliefs, foods, media, and people.
- Low-vibration emotions like resentment, guilt, fear, shame, hate, and regret.
- Not living in alignment with your truth.
- Overstimulation.
- Not being present.

Amplify the practices and environments in your life that charge your batteries:

- Habits that support your hardware, such as drinking clean water, eating live foods; getting sunlight, exercise, and deep sleep; and spending time grounding and connecting with nature.
- High-vibration feelings and actions that bring you love, joy, and happiness.
- Connection to others who raise your vibration.
- Being in service to others in need.
- Channeling energy from the infinite source—the spirit— through intention, breathwork, and meditative practices.
- Plant medicine when needed.
- Carrying positive emotions with you from moment to moment, and remembering you have the option to choose your attitude.

You are in control of how you treat your hardware, as well as the software you download and the programs you run. When you awaken and realize that those old programs don't align with who you truly are, you will no longer be a victim;

you will be able to control your destiny. Your software can be reprogrammed as you create new habits to bring your system back to nature.

NEW PROGRAMMING

When you were a child, your conscious mind was like an empty iPod with no music on it, and over time, the things that you saw and heard were songs that you downloaded. What song do you want playing? The song your father, teacher, or the media programmed? Or the song *you* want programmed?

Many times, people think they have a hardware issue when they're really dealing with a software problem. For example, inflammation can be from a negative programming such as always feeling frustrated by your environment. So how do we upgrade the subconscious?

The great news is, you can reprogram your software through repetition—the same way the original programming was put in place. If you think bad thoughts, you learned them through repetition. If you wake up feeling like crap, you learned that through repetition, either from a lifestyle that is damaging to your hardware or from childhood patterns. The first step to reversing this software is to recognize you have a habit you do not like. And the second step is to take action and create a new habit.

For example, if someone just puts one foot in front of the other to get to the gym every day, after a while it will become a habit. At first it will be tough but then it will natural and automatic.

For example, if you want to lose weight, the first step is just showing up to the gym consistently. It can be tough at first to put one foot in front of the other to get there, but with enough repetition it will become natural and automatic. Think of how you learned to drive: you never had a program for driving as a little kid nor is it factory installed, but through repetition you got better and better at it until now, as an adult, you can drive to a familiar place on autopilot. This is because your brain is an amazing machine. When you first learn a new skill, the prefrontal cortex, the conscious part of the mind, has to work through it. When you're creating a new habit of going to the gym, you will have to deal with the thoughts that pop up in your mind for why you shouldn't go and how difficult it is to get out of bed. But with repetition, the brain has this awesome power to transfer the skill to another part of the brain that doesn't take conscious thought. It then frees up the prefrontal cortex for other thinking tasks. It allows you to drive and think about other things rather than just focusing on the road.

About 97 percent of the population will only read about how they could take steps to improve their health, but won't do take any action. Become a 3 percenter: use the hacks in this book to create new habits. The efforts you make to bring your body and your spirit back to nature can have major positive effects on not only you and your health but loved ones and the community around you.

THE BODY AUTOMATICALLY HEALS

The body is a miracle. It constantly takes care of us in ways we're not even fully conscious of—it manages every single process, down to every single cell. Our bodies are constantly healing.

If you ever need a reminder of your body's incredible capacity to thrive, just remember that as you sat in your mother's womb, you grew from nothing into the person you are. Isn't that in itself a miracle? Then you were born and you were in a state of complete surrender: you had no control, and the world took care of you the best it could—and if you believe it didn't, you have the power to change that story and even accept that the circumstances of your life were necessary for you to become who you are.

Acceptance is an incredibly powerful tool in any healing journey. I ran my body into the ground because I refused to accept that I was sick and needed rest. I was trying to let my ego run the show. I was making myself perform through sheer will. I fought through everything. It was only when I began to surrender or align my will with nature's will or God's will that I began to get well. You can't fight an autoimmune disease—the disease is the body fighting itself. Instead, you can accept where you are, pay attention to what your body needs, and take action to cleanse your body and support it with the environment and practices it needs.

Carl Jung famously said that what we resist persists. When you attend to your body's needs and trust your body to heal itself, your body will begin to open up. Energy will flow more freely. That's when true transformation happens.

If you sat down to read this book in a state of dis-ease, you now know where to begin. You can't heal in the environment that made you sick. You can develop awareness of the effects your internal and external environment has on you, and you can make changes: you can get out in nature, move more, eat fresh live foods, remove toxins, and spend time around people that raise your frequency and consciousness. You can also develop awareness of your internal environment, and cultivate the thoughts, feelings, and beliefs that raise your energy.

On a daily basis, take an inventory of your environment. What are the things that make you feel fearful, angry, frustrated, guilty, or shamed? Rate them as positive, negative, or neutral. In what ways can you remove the negative? If you can't remove those environmental factors, how can you create acceptance for them and shift the feelings and stories you have around those influences? Then notice: what are the things that make you feel peace, joy, happiness, and love? How can you spend more time with those influences? How can you allow those feelings to permeate your awareness?

All of the practices in this book are designed to help you raise your consciousness and connect to your body and to nature since you are nature. The most powerful thing you can do for your health is to begin to experiment with these hacks and see what feels good to you.

Above all, trust your body to heal. When you listen to your intuition, your true nature will guide you to what is right for you and your body.

Through my EarthFIT training facilities and my Back Pain Relief 4 Life program, I'm surrounded by a community of people who are taking their healing journeys together. Visit each of these communities online to find additional resources and connect with others who are putting these hacks in practice to heal:

- Healing Hacks: healinghacks.net
- EarthFIT: earthfittraining.com https://www.facebook.com/EarthFITTrainingFacility/
- Back Pain Relief4Life: backpainrelief4life.com https://www.facebook.com/MyBackPainCoach/

Come share your own journey as you reconnect with your soul's calling and bring your body back to nature.

APPENDIX

SIMPLE METHOD GUARANTEED TO HELP STIMULATE THE HEALING PROCESS

Throughout this book, we've discussed many hacks and habits to help the body heal. If you're just beginning your healing journey, it can be overwhelming to know where to start—but here's a quick summary of the simple steps you can take to bring your body back to nature.

STEP ONE: REMOVE TOXINS, POISONS, AND INFLAMERS

Remove the following foods from your diet:

- Grains (especially wheat)
- Processed dairy
- Conventional processed meats
- Alcohol
- Refined sugars
- GMO products
- Pesticides
- Soy products (except fermented soy)

- Junk food and packaged processed foods, especially those containing dyes, additives, or corn syrup

Remove the following toxic products from your home and environment:

- Nonstick pans (Use cast iron, ceramic, or glass)
- Fabric softeners
- Air fresheners
- Aerosols and detergents for both clothing and dishes
- Shampoos and conditioners, hair dyes
- Pesticides
- Bug spray with Deet
- Commercial sunblocks
- Beauty products
- Amalgam fillings
- Jewelry that contains toxic heavy metals

Remove the thoughts that made you sick:

- Take inventory of when you feel judgement, guilt, shame, anger, and other negative emotions.
- As much as possible, remove the triggers for negative emotions.
- Make a daily practice of giving yourself positive affirmations and expressing gratitude.

STEP TWO: RENOURISH

Increase your fruit and veggie consumption:

- Blend fruits and if you have gut damage, juice veggies. If your gut can handle vegetable fiber, juice both.

- Get lots of greens.

Start with intermittent fasting a few times a week:

- Eat your meals in an eight-hour window, fasting for sixteen hours.

Increase your oxygen consumption:

- Incorporate breathwork, such as the Wim Hof Method (low cost).
- Spend time in a hyperbaric oxygen chamber (higher cost).
- Exercise, focusing on rebounding, jogging, and activities that help you sweat and move the lymph.
- Spend time in a hypobaric oxygen chamber (CVAC).

Spend time in nature:

- Get sunlight to boost your vitamin D levels.
- Connect with the earth through grounding.
- Meditate.

STEP THREE: REPAIR AND REBOOT

Start with easy cleanses, such as castor oil packs:

- Put on a castor oil pack every night for one week to start, and more if you need it.

Take steps to detox:

- Use an infrared sauna.

- Use PEMF, such as the AmpCoil or Biocharger, to increase cellular function and reharmonize organs and tissues.
- Do enemas at home, or consult a professional for colonics.
- Use binders to process out toxins (remember to always consult a professional before heavy metal detoxing).

Boost your neuroplasticity:

- Use psychedelics if you feel it is necessary and it calls to you.

Continue the benefits:

- Twice a year, do a three- to five-day water fast or juicing fast.

As you experience healing with this simple method, you can return to the individual chapters for additional hacks to boost your practice. You are your most important science experiment: try these steps and pay attention to how you feel. Find what recharges your batteries and brings you back to nature and vibrant health.

ACKNOWLEDGMENTS

I would like to acknowledge all the true healers who have sacrificed their time, energy, and sometimes their lives and careers; who didn't compromise their morals and integrity on the journey to provide root-level relief and healing for others. True healers are committed to the truth and sharing it with the world with pure, good intentions and love without fear, backlash, or retribution.

ABOUT THE AUTHOR

IAN HART is a fitness expert who has dedicated his life and his career to helping others heal naturally. He's the owner of Back Pain Relief4Life—the simplest and most effective way to eliminate back pain naturally and fast—and the co-founder of My Back Pain Coach. He is also the creator of EarthFIT Training Systems and owns and operates a top-rated training facility with three locations. Ian's work has been featured in *Men's Health Magazine,* and he's appeared as a health expert on *New York 1 News.* In addition to his work, Ian also hosts regular wellness retreats in the Costa Rican rainforest.

Lightning Source UK Ltd.
Milton Keynes UK
UKHW011023250520
363829UK00001B/37/J